HEALTH & POWER

HEALTH & POWER

Learn how to delete illness, pain and suffering using key Energy Testing Tools to discover the facts from your own body.

———

Andrea Smith Banks, B.F.A.

Cover Design by Andrea Smith Banks

ISBN: 0974495905
ISBN 13: 9780974495903

Disclaimer

The information in HEALTH & POWER is for educational purposes only and is based solely on my personal experience, studies, and conclusions. If you have a medical problem please seek proper professional help. I am not responsible or liable in any way to readers or others for the way they use my educational information in this book. I am not a doctor.

Andrea Smith Banks

Dedication

This book is dedicated to Dr. Susan Godman, ND, without whose help I wouldn't be here to write it. Her love and guidance helped me through my darkest hours. I also want to thank my brother Edward J. Smith, Jr., who has been in my corner since birth, and whose love magnifies my spirit.

Contents

Preface

I'm writing my story—how I took back my health and power by knowing how to determine the truth behind my illness and understanding the powerful energy our bodies need to heal. I want you to take the shortcuts in this book and benefit from the lessons I learned the long, hard way. When I got so fatigued that I spent the better part of ten years in bed, I managed my commercial real estate only on my "good" days. Back then, I had two little dogs that needed to be fed, and on my "bad" days, feeding them was all I could do. If I hadn't been committed to their love, I would really have been committed! I'm sure you each know pain and suffering well or have others close to you who do, but not having enough energy to get five feet to the bathroom? Climbing up the two flights of stairs on my elbows because my knees and hips became paralyzed? I mean, even body odor left me. I kept it all to myself, and nobody could understand those years of isolation. No allopathic MDs could discover what was wrong with me, yet all agreed I was out of luck. I looked in the mirror and saw the "walking dead," so I stopped looking.

Then came a holistic health fair where I found "alternative" healers, and I started getting answers. I had gone to three separate shrinks before that; they had kept me on drugs that made me comatose for five years while I gained fifty pounds. At this holistic health fair, I learned about having mercury poisoning from the fillings in my teeth. One healer pricked my finger and isolated a red blood cell that was encircled with a thick, gray rim, which indicated heavy metals. He asked me if I ate a lot of fish, too, and the sicker I got the more Swordfish I ate, loaded with mercury as I learned later. Another Chinese doctor I saw at this fair looked at my tongue and fingernails and told me the same thing. Not one MD practicing Western medicine or any of the four psychiatrists I saw had ever asked me if I had a lot of fillings in my teeth. Luckily, alternative medical practices look for the cause of the problem so that a cure can be found. Western medicine usually only treats symptoms, not the whole body or causes.

I finally got news I could use, and I read all about Hal Huggins, the former DDS whose license was taken away for blowing the whistle on mercury poisoning from amalgam fillings (silver fillings). His book *It's All in your Head* was recommended to me and I finally "got it". I was tested for heavy metals and had the highest number the Nevada Clinic had ever seen. At last, I came out of my isolation and let go of my feelings of dejection and rejection. I had found these new natural healers—holistic MDs, naturopaths, chiropractors, and so on—who understood that I was not a hypochondriac and that it wasn't "all in my head." My fatigued, slow-motion life was real and understood by these people. I had never known about holistic anything before that, or natural healing, as there is no fortune to be made by them via patents and marketing. So I now saw a whole new picture. I had finally found the truth, and it really did set me free. This book tells you how you can achieve this, too.

At that time, hardly any information about Lyme disease was available, so when I later bought my fantastic biofeedback machine, the EPFX/SCIO, which tests one's body frequency against the frequencies of over ten thousand illnesses, allopathic treatments, Chinese medicine, natural supplements, and so on, Lyme kept coming up for me in high numbers. I was also reading the *Townsend Letter*, and Lyme and its coinfections just began to appear. So my new biofeedback machine, which is based on quantum physics, diagnosed me when all the western allopathic doctors I'd seen all my life couldn't. I realized that I had been bitten by everything in the forests since I was two years old, and now that I was in my fifties, I finally had an answer.

Whether you have Lyme or chronic illness or MS or whatever, I found the very best tools you can use to find the truth, to get true answers, plus books you will find helpful. I tell you exactly how they worked for me, allowing me to take back the health and the power I'd lost as a victim of medical ignorance. I turned my chronic fatigue into a memory, and I am healthier today in my seventies than I ever was, even as a child. I manage my health day by day using the tools of truth, kinesiology, Dowsing, and the internationally famous "Map of Consciousness" devised by David Hawkins, MD, in his incredible book *Power vs. Force*. You will also read about other truth tools that I use.

In a conversational style, I talk about the truth that is essential to me after all the rejection and loneliness and how I built an all-new foundation for myself using these truth tools and techniques to advise me. The spiritual path they created for me is thanks to the greatest givers: His Holiness the Buddha Maitreya (Maitreya means teacher) (www.buddhamaitreyahealingtools.com,), the indefatigable Oprah and her Super Soul Sundays, and Dr. Rev. Michael Bernard Beckwith, who created the incredible Agape International Spiritual Center, and his talented wife, Rickie Byars Beckwith, the spiritually gifted musician and songwriter. Rickie amplifies the spiritual truth out loud on the CDs of the Agape Services that I subscribe to weekly and listen to daily in my car. God bless the givers. They supported me, and from the truth tools and truth heroes I discuss, I learned that the truth does set you free, over and over.

I hope that the truth tools in Chapter One deliver a new power you can use to guide your healing and health, because with them you can't make mistakes anymore and can't be misled or manipulated. It will be as if you are now and forevermore on top of your mountain with an overview of the rest of the world that is honest and real.

I chased freedom like a maniac all my life, and even though I had ninety-five percent more freedom than anyone else, I never felt free. That's because I never felt "well." I couldn't count on myself to make plans for the future because I didn't know how I would feel next week, or even tomorrow. I became more and more isolated, because Lymees get tired of their own "story" after a while. I joked that I could see why people steal the identities of others. I was sick of my own story and wanted to walk away from myself! I used Bowen Therapy and my Richway Biomat for my awful muscle spasms and tension, so I didn't have to drink wine for relief from Pyroluria and the anxiety it created physically along with Lyme and all it's coin-fections. No two days were the same, ever, and I never knew what tomorrow's symptoms or energy level or mood was going to be. Pyrroles double under stress, and my entire life was stressful—from my childhood to my real estate investment business to my professional art business. My biofeedback machine was the only friend I had, besides my wonderful naturopath doctor. I used Rolfing to help my back and walking, got chiropractic adjustments as needed, and used Bowen, Theta Healing, and so on when my spine collapsed and with it my posture.

I did meditation and nature walks, but my Naturopathic Doctor Susan Godman was my rock from fifteen years ago. She is an angel and a genius, and she has been a true friend as well as the best doctor I ever had. I never knew alternative medicine existed before I met her in Arizona, and she kept me alive during my "walking dead" period, before we knew I had Lyme. I used Phyllis A. Balch's *Prescription* for *Nutritional Healing* as one guide book, and then came the stores Whole Foods, Sprouts, Natural Grocers, and others that carried organic food and supplements. Thank God.

I always took responsibility for my illness. Even though we may feel like victims, I knew that spiritually everyone is responsible for whatever happens to them, as they are on the plane and energetic frequency that attracted it. I found Dr. Arthur Janov's great 1973 book, *Primal Man: The New Consciousness*, at a library sale when I lived in Laguna Beach. He wrote a gold classic, talking about the childhood injuries that create the roots of neuroses that follow us for life. We develop a personality around the primal pain source to protect it, and it will be with us for life unless we identify it and release it. I saw my personality as totally made up to please others. Having a screaming mother, I became a "people pleaser" (the book *The Disease to Please* by Harriet Braiker was great). I was putting my pseudo personality out there to get ahead, to make people like me, love me, and accept me. But there was no me. I lived on "shoulds, musts, and oughts," as anyone who has had therapy as long as I did knows very well.

My dear father, the inventor and composer, died when I was twelve and left me alone with my mother, who throughout my life preferred my year-older brother. So in order to get somewhere, I kept adding layers of new personality to my core. I was like a cardboard cutout, going to modeling school, working as a bunny for Playboy in New York, and smiling at everyone I was supposed to smile at. When I was home alone, I would read every book I could and think, think, think. (When I was in high school and on the honor roll, my mother would scream at me to "think, think, think," so when I wasn't living with her anymore, I said it for her.) While on campus, at lectures, and reading, I always felt good learning. All my life I thought I was supposed to be here as a witness. To this day, I don't know why. I do know that in four years at Syracuse University to receive my BFA, I had no connection to anybody but my boyfriend, whom I later married. The teacher whose department I was in for my Fashion Illustration class hated me (she had good looks but a disabled leg) for all four years, and several of the male teachers were trying to enamor me, as were several other older boys on campus. It was so cold, and I was very unhappy, but my mother said, "You never finish anything!" So I resisted the temptation to go back to the Big Apple where I belonged. All artists start with stressed out childhoods, it's a given, so I had talent to spare all my life.

I also had abandonment issues as well as suppressed grief and pain issues, hence became a perfectionist and a workaholic, my wounded heart trying to avoid feeling. I stayed inside my head, as all the therapists later told me. The book *Paradox and Healing* by Dr. Michael Greenwood and Dr. Peter Nunn is worth reading, as they show how none of us go unscathed through our earliest years. My mother and I even had different Rh factors in our type O blood: I was negative and she was positive, so we were fated right from the start. (This doesn't happen with firstborn children, so my brother was fine.)

The book *Love Your Disease* by John Harrison, MD, really helped me see how childhood beliefs are made early and are acted out for the rest of our lives. This reminds me of Dr. Ryke Hamer's learning how the brain records the unexpected and unresolved dramatic shock to spare us from the strong stress hormones that could kill us and puts the event in storage to resolve or address later, which can cause illness if not remedied. We should be thankful for this, which is the same as loving your disease. *Biogeneology Sourcebook: Healing the Body by Resolving Traumas of the Past* by Christian Niche discusses Dr. Hamer's discoveries and how to use them to heal. I will talk about Dr. Hamer later along with other truth heroes. But for now, think about all the truth tools I used to find out all about these things, without another therapist, by asking a ton of questions and keeping a journal for the answers. You will be amazed how you will learn who you really are and be able to see through the pseudo you that it was necessary to create for the child you are protecting and the illness it caused.

What really thrilled me was the machine. The biofeedback machine caught me every time I wasn't being truthful, giving me notes indicating that I was "bargaining," for example. I would say, "What?" But the more I thought about what it meant, the more I realized it was right. It was like being invaded without permission, but I needed it in order to learn about my real self. Sometimes "greed" came up, for instance, and I would then think through the things in my life that would apply, and it was clear. It said to me over and over again at the beginning that I was not willing to change or was unaware. Boy, did that make me mad, even when I thought I was "getting it!" This machine, based on principles of quantum physics, was so far above everything I had ever read or known and so complex that it was hard, even with all the extensive training I took for it in Puerto Vallarta, Budapest, Santa Monica, and at home with the brilliant Dr. Debbie Drake's DVDs, and all the other great teachers, including the genius inventor, Professor Bill Nelson. I feel as if I have done years of graduate work in best information center of any, the EPFX/SCIO, in the fourteen years I've had the machine after purchasing it from Canada. I learn so much each week I use it, available nowhere else, based on the truth.

The Rife frequencies are all in the EPFX/SCIO, Dr. Hamer's work, allopathic cures, supplements, vitamin deficiencies, allergies, emotional blocks, mental blocks, energy levels, all the pathogens to zap, color therapy, meridians, polarity...I could go on and on. This addition to my health studies was formidable in my education about health, and continues every time I use it. I have my health dictionary on hand each time, and I learn even more, so it's as if I had lessons every week for fourteen years in addition to all the books I've read. I find it totally fascinating, because quantum physics is totally fascinating. My body and mind are inspired, and my spirit, my thoughts, my beliefs—all are in frequencies on the EPFX/SCIO. Thank you, Professor Nelson. I have mentioned him in other places in the book, but I can't say enough about this genius. Did I mention that this inventor brought the astronauts back from the spaceship when the rest of the scientists in charge couldn't get them home? Look it up online.

I met my match with this machine. Computer based, this small box of genius, attached to a laptop, taught me so many things I would never have learned anywhere else in the linear education of Western medicine. Because it was holistic, based on quantum physics, and included everything out there, including electroacupuncture, homeopathy, Chinese medicine, and so much more, this frequency testing in subspace can test people far away from it physically. My clients are amazed by the things that come up in their testing even if they don't tell me of their past conditions, it all comes out in numbers on the machine. I use the machine for my own treatments once a week, twice a week if I want to do more, and it saved me from being one of the "walking dead." It gave me my life back, as did the other truth tools I will introduce to you that were also instrumental in my taking back my health and my power, and becoming free at last.

I know these truth tools will help each and every one of you, and practicing them will reduce and eliminate your days of pain and suffering a lot faster than all the years it took me to find them and apply their light of truth. I would love to hear your stories about how these tools are working for you. I am available as a Consultant and Biofeedback Practitioner via my website: www.

andreabanksartsandbooks.com, so please access the "Contact" link and drop me a line. You can check out my art there too.

Because the evolving pathogens like Lyme, that have been here for millions of years are epidemic now, we need to become our own healers and Medical Detectives to turn our negatives into positives. Using these tools, you will find the truths you need to make intelligent decisions about your health. And if it makes you angry at first, good. Because there's a lot of energy in that anger—energy that you can transform to get well. That anger will turn to gratitude as you begin to feel better and better. I realized that for most of my life, I was sicker than I knew, because as I got better, I realized that I'd never felt so good before. I was amazed, since I thought everybody felt the way I did. So it was the truth that set me free, and I hope each one of you who reads this book will find that freedom too and feel the gratitude as you heal your body, mind, and spirit.

Introduction

I was just two and my big brother was three in our first encounter with the law. The newspapers wrote it up that we were lost, but I knew my big brother, and he was never lost. That's why I always followed him. So a year later, when we did it again and the cops found us, the newspaper headline was, "They're off again!" We were three and four then, and we felt very inconvenienced by being delivered back home. Mom never reprimanded us, anyway. As we ran off into the woods every day to explore and play like feral children, she'd never ask us where we went.

My year older brother, Eddy, was the whole horizon to me, the back of his red flannel shirt all I could see. I stayed close so I wouldn't get lost, or eaten. The sounds of the forest were musical, and all the animals but us spoke or yakked or sang. We moved from Pennsylvania to New Jersey that year, to new forests and sounds, and we were excited to see the new territory. This time we had cows to ride in a big pasture. Eddy named the Butterfly Forest, the Big Forest, the Little Forest, and we ate berries and played with pollywogs. We never had to speak a word to enjoy our feral lifestyle. We only went home when it was getting dark and we got hungry. Eddy always remembered the way home even if we were miles away, and I trusted him to keep me safe, especially after he pulled me out of quicksand once and another time sawed me out of a tree. That was life—until school got in the way, and then we had to wait for the weekends to go back into the forest. This lasted until we were ten and eleven, as I recall.

The only downside of our life outdoors was that everything bit me, and I mean everything that could fly or crawl had me for lunch and dinner from the age of two onward. Not Eddy—he'd only get a bite here and there. New Jersey mosquitos looked big enough to be aircraft to me, and they sucked deep and long, leaving big welts all over me. But back then, it didn't seem to matter.

What I learned much later was that they were injecting me with Lyme disease, Ehrlichia, Brucellosis, Bartonella, Mycoplasma, Babesia (like Malaria), molds, Herpes, Epstein-Barr virus (EBV), and more. I was a major bug attractor all my life, and I learned much later that people with a vitamin B deficiency attract bugs most. Stress is a big user of B vitamins, and ultimately the stress caused by the body's trying to fight all these infections is enormous and eventually wears out even the strongest immune system. This is what happened to me.

On and off through my very exciting life, I was sick and had on-and-off low energy and various symptoms, but no MDs could find anything wrong, eventually saying, "It's all in your head!" You've heard that before. Binge drinking wine made me feel better and probably killed off enough bugs through drowning in alcohol, which worked as a reset for me.

There were many episodes of illness that I mixed with owning real estate in Las Vegas—talk about stressors! I owned twenty-eight apartment units for twenty-eight years. Since I never had to answer to anybody else, I just kept my illness to myself until I was in my fifties, when my immune system walked off the job. I started enduring some serious pain and suffering and some enormously lengthy fatigue. Again, no MDs could help. It was only when I stumbled into that holistic health fair and learned that alternative medicine, or holistic or integrative medicine, existed that things turned around. By then I was the "walking dead," and everyone thought I was going to die, including me. That was about fifteen years ago.

Fourteen years ago, as I mentioned, I bought the biofeedback machine based on quantum physics, and I finally found through the results of testing with it that I had Lyme disease and many of it's coinfections, that get injected by ticks, mosquitos, flies, anything that bites. This fabulous machine gave me one of the biggest "aha" moments ever when I found that the truth was "holographic", or three-dimensional. No wonder all of linear allopathic/Western medicine got stuck in the dark ages of linear or two-dimensional thinking, compared to alternative methods, like energy medicine, like biofeedback, and so on. Even Dr. Oz said, "Energy medicine is the medicine of the future." The future is now.

My personal search for my health took years, and the discoveries I made over these years include the truth tools I found in my struggle with chronic illness. I am very happy to pass these on to you. Since I am also an empath and can feel all the pain and suffering that others feel, we both gain.

Besides, today I am healthier than I ever remember being because of how these truth tools have set me free. I am no longer at the mercy of the ill-educated MDs or other teachings, and my core is based on the new paradigm of the truth and nothing but the truth, which my tools provide for as truth guides.

I will be talking about taking back your health and your power. In Chapter Two the incredible books I mention meant so much to turning me to the truth, like *Power vs. Force* by Dr. David Hawkins. This book should be taught in every school in the world today. His famous "Map of Consciousness" first described in *Power vs. Force* is used worldwide today, as it shows us how to calibrate the truthfulness or falsehood of anything and everything via kinesiology, which I'll explain shortly.

If our leaders were aware of the difference in the levels of consciousness of people like terrorists, they would see that the very title *Power vs. Force* shows that "force" can never be successful because every time force is used, there is retaliation of force back. Learning about real "power" is the answer, as is raising your level of consciousness. Ghandi used power, not force.

Power vs. Force changed my life, and it came out years ago. I have seen some fantastic books disappear over time and be forgotten. Since Dr. Hawkins passed on and no longer lectures in Sedona (luckily his lectures are on DVDs with Veritas Publishing), I fear that present and future generations will miss what may be the most important lessons of truth in their lives. Dr. Hawkins shows how, when you raise the level of your own consciousness, you can also raise the levels of millions of others with you simultaneously around the globe. In my opinion, Dr. Hawkins stands on the highest chair of perception.

It took Dr. Hawkins ten years to write this book in order to get each chapter over 700 on his Map of Consciousness ratings from 0 to 1,000. (I just tested Eckhart Tolle's popular book *Power of Now* and got only 450. I was surprised because I liked it so much, but figured that it was because it was about "time", a man-made construct, so very superficial to intrinsic value.) You can see that since 700 is also the level of Gandhi, and 1,000, the highest, is the level of the original words of Jesus or of Buddha, hence *Power vs. Force* is in the best company for consciousness and truthfulness. You will learn how to use the Map of Consciousness by reading my book, and you can check these results yourself using these truth tools. This testing, using kinesiology, and the tools of truth, allowed me to find the truth about my health, books, politicians, drugs, doctors, tests, friendships, and everything else through numerical calibration using this incredible resource. Energy is in everything, and IS everything, Source, God, as you like, so what tests can be better than Energy tests?

My testimony here is from my own experience, and I have nothing to lose telling the whole truth and nothing but the truth. I will mention many more tools that are from top books, people, methods, and so on, all of which you can find for yourself by checking into them and then throwing away pain and suffering like a bad habit. I recently heard an MD say on TV that over one hundred million Americans suffer from chronic pain. I was amazed, because if you exclude kids, that's half the population of the country. And we wonder why heroin is such an incredible problem in every age group today?

So, one of my suggestions in the following pages is to say no to drugs again, but now it means *all* drugs, *any* drugs. Let's mark them "in case of emergency only." I know how you feel seeing their ads on TV. I feel the same way. They know that via repetition, eventually the public will just accept that some of the drugs can even cause death, and that's fine, as "side effects" are fine too. I feel used, lied to, manipulated and outgunned, but this too will pass when we take our power back and say no to drugs, even over the counter ones, because there are natural remedies for nearly everything. I just didn't know about them before my illness because they didn't have any TV time or advertising. Little by little I learned about them and saw the difference they made, without side effects.

We're going to change all that by using the truth tools in this book, saying no to drugs by the millions as we learn the truth about why we are feeling this pain, using natural healers, checking out the food supply, and eating organically. We will gain strength quickly, and take more giant steps as we learn who we are. We will fall in love with ourselves all over again by walking into the new paradigm of the truth and nothing but the truth. The new paradigm will restore your faith as you constantly test information you're being told or that you read or hear on TV or the radio or online. I actually stopped listening to the "opinions" out there, friends and family included, because I could use my truth tools for the best answers of all, all the time. I have seen from my biofeedback experience that we are each different and must do different things for health—there is no one health protocol that fits all. For example, I used to "eat greens" until I learned that lectins are highest in greens and tomatoes. Flax oil is another, since people with northern European ancestry are usually allergic to it, like I am. Now the rage is coconut oil, but unless you were born where palm trees live, you may be allergic to that too. I was born in the northeastern United States of Northern European ancestry, and am allergic to coconut. What about you? Just ask your truth tools and learn about your food allergies or temporary sensitivities., a big influence on healing.

Most of the information in this book will be new to you. I learned all these things through years of extensive research and kinesiology testing, using my fantastic truth tools over many years of former trial and error. Using these same tools that I am going to teach you about, you can verify for yourself the truthfulness of everything I'm saying in this book. How's that for verification?

HEALTH & POWER is for absolutely everyone because these tools are a lifelong asset. They may be used preventatively, in all your choices in life, to be sure that you're working in your own best interest via simple yes and no answers to your questions. Life became so simple for me after I found these truth tools, and I took my life back from all those out there trying to influence me every minute. I learned to trust again. Self-doubt disappeared for good. Even my posture improved along with my confidence.

Today, I feel so grateful that I stayed on the spiritual path that only appeared through illness, where I found the truth tools my pain and suffering showed me. I am a much better person after the long journey, and it makes me happy to give you the shortcuts to taking back your own health and power. So, let's get started!

CHAPTER 1

Truth Tools

I found these truth tools over a period of years, and they are the most important pieces of information in *HEALTH & POWER*, as they are the truth finders that will set you free. I talk about six things:

1. The Map of Consciousness from *Power vs. Force* by Dr. David Hawkins, MD, calibrating values of anything you want to test, be it books, people, teachers, etc.
2. Kinesiology now uses several forms for energy testing, like arm testing.
3. Dowsing tools for Energy testing, like pendulums, rods, etc.
4. Yuen Method -Dr. Kam Yuen, thirty-fifth-generation Shaolin kung fu grandmaster using kinesiology as one method of energy testing.
5. Biofeedback Machine (Prof. Bill Nelson) reading Energy frequencies in the body.
6. The Syncrometer invented by Dr. Hulda Clark—for self-testing to give you answers electrically from the body's energy, and you can assemble your own economically.

These all use kinesiology testing or energy testing, and the EPFX/SCIO is frequency testing using electricity, as is the Syncrometer, but all of these are reading the body as the vehicle receiving and sending information, and the body never lies. (The mind is another story.)

I have experimented with many other things, but none could hold a candle to these truth tools, so forget other "experts." Become your own best friend who has all the right answers all the time by using these tools. Watch your self-doubt, fear, and worry dissolve. Feel your self-confidence soar, and get that feel-good high of the "aha" moments over and over again as you become your own Medical Detective and start defining your real health picture from now on—using tools you can trust to take your health back, and your power back. This is a short version of these top truth tools, you can look up online for more information:

1. The Map of Consciousness

Developed by David R. Hawkins, MD, PhD, and profiled in his book *Power vs. Force: The Hidden Determinants of Human Behavior: An Anatomy of Consciousness*, this is more of a chart than a map, and is now used worldwide to calibrate the energy level of anything and everything using kinesiology. (Dr. Hawkins used arm testing, but I also like the pendulum, as the arm test requires two people.) Simple yes/no answers can tell you whether a book is worth reading, a lab test is accurate, your MD is good for you, your friends are telling you the truth, your teachers are good, and so on.

You will find that the second chapter of *HEALTH & POWER* lists truth heroes and their books, and I calibrated these books. Calibration numbers represent a logarithmic progression, and the numbers scale is from 0 to 1,000, with numbers below 200 being destructive of life and false and those over 200 being constructive and true. Dr. Wayne W. Dyer called *Power vs. Force* "perhaps the most important and significant book I've read in the past ten years." For someone like Dyer, who read the ancient Persian sutras of Patanjali, you get the picture. I still consider *Power vs. Force* the most important book I ever read, and I've given copies to all my family members.

Dr. Hawkins's actual Map of Consciousness cannot be reproduced here due to copyright laws, but it is easy to find online—and now is a good time to do that so you will understand it, and can use it from here on to test. The Institute for Spiritual Research, Inc. (www.veritaspub.com) has a color laminated one, but for now, any will do for you to be able to follow it, which is extremely important for the rest of your lives as it is for mine! Look it up online for images of it you can print out now.

In his book, Dr. Hawkins describes how he found that people in the United States calibrated in total at over 400, and explained how only four percent of the population of the world calibrates over 400. People at 150 though, (under 200) are constantly hating everything and everybody, he points out. Remember he was a well-respected Psychiatrist in New York before writing this book over ten years isolated in a cabin in upstate New York. Understanding this via the Map of Consciousness shows how violence and its level of consciousness exist and are so difficult for us to see. I will talk more about *Power vs. Force* and Dr. Hawkins in the next chapter, but one of his main points is that we can raise the level of consciousness of millions of people simply by raising our own. From the first time, when I read this book over twenty years ago, I gave up rescuing others and still try daily to raise my own level of consciousness by calibrating books I read to be over 600. I then chose who I listen to, and—most important—my health questions, friendships, family, and even my little dog. (Is he just playing me? Is he really hungry?)

Dr. Hawkins says numbers in the 300s are for great churches, police, and firefighters; the 400s bring reason and logic; and the 500s shows the spiritual and level of love. So the haters at 150 can't become the lovers of the 500s overnight, as it takes generations to raise the level of consciousness that much. I calibrated myself at 555 now, up from 530 when I first read *Power vs. Force* over twenty years ago, so it's gradual. The low calibration haters will take generations to raise their calibrations through learning and experience. I pray for them.

At 600, time stops, and people reach bliss, and 700 is where Mahatma Gandhi calibrates. Gandhi's peace, selflessness, and ego-less practices showed his power to win over the force of the British Empire, which wanted to maintain control of India. Because they could not change him, this power led to India's freedom. Dr. Hawkins proves that "power cannot be resisted, but force can." Our political leaders should read this. He maintains that peace is there all the time and that we only have to remove the things in the way of it. Nothing is the "cause" of anything, and the cause-and-effect idea is an Ego construct of the intellect. Remember it's the body that never lies, not the mind! We need to refuse the Ego that wants everything, because once you're in duality, you can't win. By taking responsibility for the consequences of his own perceptions, Dr. Hawkins says he transcended the role of victim and anything having power over him. Hence, nothing can create stress in you but you. There goes "blame" and good riddens.

The original words of Jesus or the Buddha or Krishna calibrate at 1,000 on the Map of Consciousness. Dr. Hawkins shows how the interpretations of religions lowered their present day values, some more than others, as the interpreters of the originals changed them. We each change the world by what we become. The more kind and loving we are, the more we see beauty and love in everything. Our compassion then relieves the suffering of others, as we raise our level of consciousness.

Throughout *HEALTH & POWER*, I will be using the Map of Consciousness to calibrate things to show you how high up the truth ladder a subject is. You can verify these things yourself, which is the beauty of it all. God bless Dr. Hawkins for this fabulous tool. *Power vs. Force* is available at www.hayhouse.com and at www.veritaspub.com and www.amazon.com, used and new. I think it should become an important addition to every library, school, and university.

2. Kinesiology

This is the study of muscles and their movement, leading us into energy testing. Some forms are:

ARM TESTING

Before beginning any form, it is best to first center yourself and detach from any emotions. Have the test subject stand straight and raise his or her dominant arm straight out to the side, palm down. Tell the subject to "resist" when you put light pressure on his or her dominant wrist using just two fingers for light pressure. When you say "resist," you get the subject's normal strength reading first by pressing down. Next, ask a question of the test person. I usually start by asking if the subject's name is Harry, for instance, when it is not. I say "resist," and the subject resists, and when I press down on the subject's wrist with two fingers, his or her arm goes down easily with no control to keep it up even if they try to. Despite the subject's effort to maintain the arm out to the side, it collapses down to his or her side from anything false, negative, or non-beneficial. Then ask that question, but use the subject's real name. When you press two fingers to the subject's wrist, his or her arm will stay very strong as it is true, positive, and good for them. If you like, add an artificial-sweetener packet to the subject's other hand and perform the arm test again. The subject's arm will go down, no matter how hard he or she tries to keep it up. I usually do this in the kitchen, the subject's or mine, because it will show him or her how easy and fun it is to test for food allergies, a very important factor in illness and immunity. The first time I did this myself, I tossed out a lot of the flavor additives I kept in the refrigerator door as they were either moldy being in there too long, or had food additives or artificial ingredients. The cleaner and fresher the foods I eat, the fewer flavorings they need anyway.

You can ask the "testee" questions like, "Is there an emotional component to your illness?" If the arm stays firm, this means yes. Does the emotional component make up ten percent of the illness cause? Fifty percent? Ninety percent? Does this emotion involve the subject's relationship with _____ now? In the past? In childhood? Was this emotion from a prenatal experience in the womb? The more you read the books I profile in the second chapter, "Truth Heroes," the better questions you will think of in no time. Your awareness will increase quickly, and you'll get one "aha" moment after another as the truth unfolds effortlessly. I love doing this. It's the best toy I ever had and it will never wear out or break! Showing your friends will impress them too, and teaching others this energy-truth tool testing will spread the good news.

When *Power vs. Force* came out, ten of us got together at Unity minister Kathy Thalden's house to try to reproduce Dr.

Hawkins's findings. Her husband was a wonderful Architect. Among the ten of us, we couldn't get consistent answers, and we wondered what we were doing wrong, because we knew that Dr. Hawkins knew a lot more than we did. Kathy put her head to this and came up with the answer that finally had all ten of us getting the same results—asking this short "Intro" question before asking anything further: "From 100 percent pure light, am I clear to test on my highest level?" We were so excited.

This way, she set up "from 100 percent pure light," meaning the pure truth as pure light, "am I clear to test" (centered, clear, connected) "on my highest level," because we each have a higher and lower level of being. All infections and negatives are extremely low frequencies (ELF), and believe me, they will answer first if you don't ask this Intro question first. This brilliant introduction Kathy invented has served me well for over twenty years, and I use it every time before starting a series of questions. It's like setting up your connection and focus on the right plane to receive the true answer. Then ask the questions to follow without using it unless your focus connection is broken, like if the phone rings or you are interrupted, this Intro question should be repeated after the interruption, before you resume the other questions.

Again, if you don't use this Intro, I guarantee you will not get correct answers. I later learned that dowsers use the introduction "May I? Can I? Should I?" which essentially covers the same bases, but I prefer Kathy's Intro even when using Dowsing. After all, Dowsing is energy testing too, so let's talk about other kinesiology tools, like the pendulum, which I lovingly call "P".

PENDULUM

I found the pendulum long before I knew it was also a Dowsing tool. I think I found it in a pendulum book, and when I tested it, it worked very successfully. I didn't need a partner to test with, either, so I was hooked. A pendulum was my new best friend; it was loyal, trustworthy, honest. My new best friend! I tested everything using the pendulum, and I bought a few more so I would always have one handy in my purse, next to my reading chair, in my desk, by my computer, next to the bed. Being an artist, I even made a bunch of them, well, about two hundred of them—I tend to overdo things when I'm inspired. You can make one of your own using any small, weighted object at the end of a string or short chain four to eight inches long. Several books exist on using a pendulum, but frankly, I've never read any of them because I prefer to keep things simple. Simply "yes" or "no". I do use the great charts for pendulums in books though, they are very help-ful and can be fast answers to vitamin deficiencies, etc. So, be clear, centered, and without emotion for the testing and you're good to go. I don't put my hand on the testee's shoul-der, as some people do when arm testing another, as I feel I could be contaminating them with my energy.

If you are using the pendulum, say the Intro, and ask a yes-or-no question while holding the pendulum about four inches from the weighted-object end, on the chain or string. Don't try to be still so as not to influence its answer—feel free to start it swinging yourself, as it will take over. If you like, you can put your elbow on the table if you are seated. A yes answer moves up and back as if you were nodding your head in the affirmative yes, and a no answer moves left to right as if you were shaking your head or watching a tennis match.

Although dowsers say to program your own pendulum, I just use the above to keep it simple, nodding up and down, right and left. I program my own focus, clearing myself of extraneous energies and emotions before I ask, and always start with the Intro.

If the pendulum won't take off, which rarely occurs, your "polarity" could be off, so just tap the lower back of your head with your hand, and try again. And if you have already asked a question, and the pendulum is not responding definitively, the answer can be a " maybe", but this is unusual. You will see big swings for yes or no answers that are strongest and most definite, like it's yelling the answer! Like taking piano lessons, practice, practice, practice! It becomes easy quickly, so hurry up and start so you can use this wonderful energy truth tool to calibrate numbers for the Map of Consciousness, Dowsing, and the Yuen Method.

Finger Circles

This is another method to use if you don't have a pendulum or a partner. Put your thumb and forefinger of each of your hands together, joined together in a figure eight formation. Ask a yes-or-no question, and if it's true or the answer is yes, your fingers will stay strongly locked in together in the eight. If the answer is no, they will slip out of being locked and will separate easily. Don't forget the Intro for each of these.

Breath

This is one of my favorites, because you only have to ask a question after the Intro and then just inhale. If the answer is

yes, your head will bend back at the neck so that you're looking at the ceiling or the sky. If the answer is no, your head
will remain rigid as you inhale. How simple! I learned this
one at the Verde Valley Dowsers meetings in Sedona years
ago, and love it because I don't need any tools beside me.

LEANING FORWARD OR BACK
This is similar except that your whole body will lean forward
for yes or backward for no after inhaling and asking the intro
and the question. Just don't fall over.

Before moving on to Dowsing, which was covered partly above in
kinesiology, I want to tell you how to use a pendulum to remove
negative or nonbeneficial energies and how to replace that negative
energy with the same amount of positive energy. Let's say you want
to get rid of your sugar cravings. First, perform the Intro, and then
start to spin the pendulum counterclockwise (to the left) in a circle.
Say, "Remove any and all desire for sugar or sweets from my body
and mind on all levels, one hundred percent present, past, and future." I use "present, past, and future" because in quantum physics,
these are all the same and could relate to past lives as well. I had a
water phobia from drowning in a past life, for instance.

The pendulum will keep going until it clears that energy and
removes it. Once it has done so, it will stop on its own. At that point,
you can ask if it was one hundred percent removed. If the answer
is yes, then you can spin the pendulum clockwise (to the right) in
a circle to replace the negative energy you removed with positive
energy. So, it's left to remove, and right to add. Then say, "Please
add the energy to my body and mind to feel satisfied about food and
content in my body, now and forever." When it stops spinning, ask

if that has been added one hundred percent. If it doesn't you can ask if there are other emotional issues behind this that you need to find?

Making these up as you go along and reading the truth heroes' books will make this another fun part of the adventure of learning the truth about who you really are. Start a group if you can and learn from each other as well. Kathy ran the *Power vs. Force* group for a whole year until we moved on. I never missed a weekly meeting; it was such fun and so empowering. Health and power go together, yes? Yes. Now, remember, no negatives allowed—no curses or death or anything like that is appropriate when using these tools. I learned not even to make any promises in this lifetime, because these promises go with you into the next life and follow you from past lives. Clearing yourself of any and all past-life contracts (poverty is a common one) or agreements is always a good idea.

3. Dowsing

Dowsing came next for me. When I moved to Prescott, Arizona, close to beautiful Sedona, with its ripples of red rocks so bright you need to wear sunglasses, I found out about the wonderful monthly Dowsing meetings held there. I learned for the first time after five years of using my pendulum that it was also a Dowsing tool! Except that as I mentioned, the dowsers say, "May I? Can I? Should I?" as opposed to our Intro: "From one hundred percent pure light, am I clear to test on my highest level?" I went to a lot of lectures at the Sedona Life Center, but none beat the Verde Valley Dowsers chapter meetings at St. Andrew's Episcopal Church, where about fifty to seventy dowsers show up monthly to hear the best speakers on new and different Dowsing techniques. I also joined The American Society of Dowsers.

I like people who love quantum physics and energy and consciousness, and I find such folks at Dowsing meetings. If you can locate a dowsers group near you, go to its meetings several times, and you will get the best education about how it all works. In Sedona, professional dowsers are paid for their work by developers who want them to find water sources in the Arizona desert, prospectors seeking gold to mine, individuals looking for people who are lost, and so on. The Verde Valley chapter sells CDs about Dowsing by different experts and speakers as well as pendulums and books. Then I found Raymon Grace, whose DVD just blew me away. Watching him play with his pendulum was eye-opening. I found that his Ozark dowsers and the Toronto dowsers joined up to save many lives in Africa and around the world by teaching them how to dowse and purify their water. It was contaminated water that spread AIDS and killed so many. Then I found Susan Collins from Canada, who also has a lot of online books and protocols and different slants on Dowsing that are quite remarkable. She was head of the Canadian Dowsers.

Other Dowsing tools exist besides the pendulum—rods, bobbers, V-rods, W-rods, Y-rods, and so on. You can use *The Dowser's Workbook* by Tom Graves to learn about them all, but it is mainly what you are trying to find out that determines what tools to use. The rods, for example, are great for covering a lot of territory, as these are held one in each hand and will stay parallel to each other and the ground until the clear energy under you isn't clear anymore. At that point, they will cross. This is good for finding Geopathic Stress and other Ley Lines and grids natural to the entire planet that can be bad for your health. I talk about this elsewhere in the book, and without a Dowsing tool, you will never know where they are. Finding any Geopathic Stressors in your home or work environment is essential, as is using Orgone pyramids or other tech tools to control their effects on your health or moving the bed or easy chair that is sitting in one. I talk about these elsewhere in this book, but the information on using Dowsing for abundance, health, clearing, raising your vibrational level, and everything else is an unbelievable power that agrees totally with quantum physics as I see it. I have witnessed many notes, one from a gal who cured herself of thyroid cancer by clearing her thyroid's life force, for example. There is no limit to the power of Dowsing tools and energy, which to me is the essence of God energy as source, as everything is energy. We only need to transform it to heal.

Within the dowsers' introduction, "May I?" asks for permission to do it, "Can I?" asks if it is possible for you to do it, and "Should I?" asks if it is a good idea for you to do it. Only universal intelligence knows. Some say that the answers to Dowsing questions come from the individual dowser's subconscious. Not in my opinion. The dowser and the tool are merely the vehicles conducting the universal energy of the answers. I believe universal truth is available out there for anyone to tap into—anytime, anywhere. That may be hard to prove, but nothing invalidates the fact that it exists and works. I find it agrees with quantum physics also. The only time it doesn't work is if you ask about the future or ask the wrong question. I used to have problems finding lost items because I forgot to say, "Where is my purse—now?" I would get yes to other locations—where it was yesterday or this morning, but not *now*. It's really fun having these learning experiences, and the more you do it, the more you will be amazed at the synchronicity. Your mind will change into a new researcher, expanding and growing, and you'll love thinking again with all your Medical Detective prowess.

I couldn't have turned my health picture around without my pendulum, that's certain. Using it to detect food allergies was really a key issue, because our immune system reacts to allergens as if each were a pathogen (the bad guys—bad bacteria, viruses, fungi) and muster all our body's energy to fight them through inflammation and calling in the immune special forces when they should be fighting the real pathogens of illness. It takes that energy to get well, and getting clear of food reactions is a big step toward health. I have found the testing done by allergy doctors totally insufficient, because my allergies are in fact really "sensitivities" that can change from one day to the next, and be caused by infectious agents, combinations, and more.

Instead of having to keep food charts of the Feingold diet, in which you don't eat the same foods for four days, I just ask "P" (recall as my nickname for the pendulum) if this is good for me now, and if P says yes, into the food cart it goes. People in the supermarket ask what I'm testing for, and I love telling them and expanding their knowledge. They love hearing about Dowsing for answers. When I open the door to the refrigerator, I ask P what to eat, and in restaurants, I run P down the menu to see what to eat there. Once I got a no to everything on the menu, so I left! Using bad oils can do serious health damage, like the oils they used there. Considering all the suffering related to having an illness, this put the fun back into my life—no kidding. And the results were spectacular. I felt back in control, taking my power back, instead of staying a victim of disease. I got stronger fast now. Health and power go together.

I could write another book about all the things I use P for. But when you see how far Dowsing can take you, you will be glad inside, because you will see the results almost weekly. Raymon Grace's books and DVDs available on his website show you how to filter your water, for example, and that includes filtering out fear and anger too, along with the spirit of greed, because you can't have the spirit of water where the spirit of greed exists, which actually characterizes all restaurants. That's just for openers. You filter out non-beneficial energies (these used to be called negative energies, but Susan Collins found that a lot of negative energy can be positive, so nonbeneficial is now the preferred term) like thought forms, fluoride, chlorine, arsenic, all chemicals, heavy metals, parasites, harmful organisms, and so on. After you ask P with a left spin to remove all the nonbeneficial energies, you then ask P if they are all gone. Raymon Grace does this over his water glass in restaurants. If the answer is yes, by spinning P to the right in a circle, it's time to add back the energy you removed, the spirit of water along with love, gratitude, vitamins, minerals, prosperity, freedom—whatever you like. Energy follows thought, so think that this thought form is immune to any nonbeneficial forces in your body, and create an ongoing matrix for yourself, as per Susan Collins books on her website, www.dowser.ca/protocolbook.html and on YouTube, which are excellent. Intent is important, so program it.

You can remove the spirit of bullying and self-punishment, as a different example, and replace the spirit of victimization and codependency with the spirit of high self-esteem, peace, unconditional love, and prosperity or whatever you need.

We are working with universal intelligence (a higher power, etc.) to remove archetypes of helplessness and other low frequencies. Scramble doubt, fear, shame, guilt, and unworthiness, neutralize negative patterns of attraction, and reprogram with a pattern of attraction to people of value. Don't put bad thought forms on yourself, like saying, "I'll be d---ed" or any self-demeaning words. We can even change the frequencies of past events and trauma. Before you start feeling overwhelmed, realize you need to get well step by step. The above is advanced Dowsing, but I want you to be aware of the depth and breadth of Dowsing today. It is no longer an old guy with a mule and a Y twig searching for water. You can take the frequency of Leukemia out of your body, for instance. The emotional causes of illness will be addressed later, but be aware that we can have a lot of subconscious negative beliefs that create interference, because your subconscious never sleeps the way your conscious mind does. Healing is about removing the interference.

Using Dowsing to detect the Ley Line energy grid all over the earth is essential, finding Geopathic Stressors that can make you ill. The American Society of Dowsers (www.dowsers.org) in Vermont may be able to find a Dowsing group near you, but you don't need one to learn. They have a lot of good books and information online, and they hold great conferences. I say start with Raymon Grace, Susan Collins, and the ASD.

4. Yuen Method

Dr. Kam Yuen was born in Hong Kong and is a thirty-fifth-generation Shaolin kung fu grandmaster. Those familiar with the *Kung Fu* television show starring David Carradine will remember Caine, the lead character, who was based on Kam Yuen. Dr.Yuen taught David Carradine the art of kung fu, and when he ran his own martial arts studios in Southern California and had film roles, he was known as the "Praying Mantis of North America."

Present-day physical therapy methods widely used in Chinese medicine have been taken directly from kung fu, and Chinese medicine is studied by kung fu men, strengthening internal organs, toning up the nerve and glandular systems, enlarging the capacity of the cardiovascular system, and strengthening skeletal muscles, all combined with deep-breathing techniques where one's diaphragm does all the work. Kung fu masters use herbal remedies numbering in the thousands.

Dr. Yuen was also a former aerospace engineer and is in the Martial Arts History Museum's Hall of Fame. World Black Belt calls him "a living legend." So, you're wondering why he's so important as a truth tool provider? Because Dr. Yuen decided that there was too much fighting in the world and that it needed more healing and less hate. He got his chiropractic license and started teaching his own instant Chinese healing, known as the Yuen Method. In this method, Dr. Yuen deletes the weaknesses in the body that cause the pain and resets the body, mind, and spirit.

Dr. Yuen uses kinesiology arm testing to demonstrate to others how he clears these weaknesses, always on the "midline" or the heart chakra, which eventually you can do without using your testing and hand movement. Dr. Yuen has been teaching his Yuen Method all over the world, and now in his seventies, he teaches in online classes or in his California studio. Kung fu taught Chinese medicine as part of kung fu, as well as herbal remedies.

I first found this incredible man when he came to Las Vegas to do a demo at the Church of Religious Science on a Thursday night. He went to other church groups also. About fifty of us were there, and Dr. Yuen asked for anyone with an illness to come up on stage with him, and a line formed. He arm-tested each person for answers, and nearly all of us went up, one after another. I remember his asking one question over and over: "Do you like the doctor you go to?" They all said yes, but each person's arm would collapse, indicating no. Remember, the body never lies. Dr. Yuen fixed every one of us that night, including me, and then signed us up for his three day all day teaching seminar that weekend. Almost all of us went, along with other church and groups, numbering hundreds for the weekend seminar.

First, Dr. Yuen showed us "toes in and toes out," where he arm-tested people's strength first with their toes turned out. They arm-tested as weak, their arms going down instead of staying firm for yes, good, positive. Then he tested them with their toes straight, and their arm tests were stronger, but were still slightly wobbly. But for those with pigeon toes, the arm tests were strongest, and their arm would stay too strong to move. What a surprise, especially because Andre Agassi was the pigeon-toed superstar in tennis at that time, and his sister Rita was my tennis coach, and she was also pigeon-toed. I felt I had finally learned their secret power!

Dr. Yuen brought us all on stage, one by one, for corrections, over the three days, and this time, well over two hundred of us received his energy healing and teachings. The way he knew what questions to ask, often regarding emotional issues, is divulged in his workbooks (levels one, two, and three) (www.yuenmethod.com) as well as his latest best seller, *Delete Pain and Stress on the Spot.*

I remember someone asking Dr. Yuen what he believed in? "Nothing," he said, "because as soon as you start defending a belief, your ego takes over, and you lose your place and awareness in the present." Ever the thirty-fifth-generation grandmaster! I use this truth as much as possible today. He said not to have likes or dislikes but to live in the now and observe, don't think. He said illness is less intense when we eliminate the effects and memories of past illnesses, of ourselves and of others, because our previous experience with sickness and the negative emotions attached to it can be triggered by a new illness, and instead of dealing with one new illness, the person suffers from hundreds or thousands of past "sickening experiences." When you eliminate the effects of the past, the present and future will be less affected, so you will hardly ever get sick, and if you do, it won't be severe and lasting. Don't feel threatened by illness, and don't dread it, or you will attract it and relive your previous illnesses. They thus become more a part of you. Be neutral about sickness, and it can last only seconds or minutes, not days and weeks. Don't take on the behavior or illness of others either—it is theirs, not ours.

I remember how I felt as I listened to Dr.Yuen's ideas and how good they made me feel. I knew they were true. The truth always makes me feel good. I calibrated Dr. Yuen's method at 1,000 on the Map of Consciousness, the highest on the scale from 1 to 1,000, the same as the original words of Jesus, Buddha, and a few others. So his teachings are true to the highest degree. I love using the Map of Consciousness to calibrate everything and anything I want to test for any reason, on any level.

So impressed with Dr. Yuen's three-day seminar, I spent the next three weeks going over his level one workbook, really learning the technique. The more specific you can be in identifying the cause of your illness or problem, and its level, the more permanent your clearing will be, and the workbooks are easy to work from. According to Dr. Yuen, if you have a pain in your shoulder, it doesn't mean it is from your shoulder. (Unfortunately, allopathic western medicine would treat only the shoulder.) Dr.Yuen says that getting the right information will disappear the problem, as they cancel each other out energetically. This is why I love it's Energetic Healing base, and how I feel it connect to Quantum Physics. Remember he was a Space Engineer, too.

I spoke with Dr. Yuen three times on the phone (yes, paid for), and he helped me enormously to get myself unstuck at different crisis times in my life. I put his Yuen Method under truth tools because it rates 1000 on the Map of Consciousness and helped me so much in my times of need.

5. EPFX/SCIO Biofeedback Machine

This computer-based machine is incredible. It is known as the EPFX in it's government registration in the USA. It is the SCIO that Dr. Nelson invented, so goes the title. It was the first to show me I had Lyme disease when dozens of western doctors couldn't. Testing over ten thousand frequencies in three minutes, yes, 10,000 frequencies in 3 minutes, the machine measures your body's responses, forming numerical answers as to which are most acute (highest) or chronic (lowest). It detects weaknesses such as viruses, nutritional deficiencies, allergies, abnormalities, and food sensitivities by calculating the biological reactivity and resonance in your body. This is testing of your energetic body and is way above and beyond most current allopathic medical tests. It measures vitamins, amino acids, minerals, enzymes, natural sugars, fatty acids, toxins, hormones, muscle tone, disease, bacteria, viruses, fungi, health of organs, detoxification, and much more. Children and animals can be treated on the machine as well. This fantastic invention has been one of the best investments I ever made. Professor Bill Nelson/Desiré Dubounet's latest upgrade is called the Eductor (www.qxsubspace.com or www.whitedovehealing.com) and any Professional Medical or Mental Health office today should have one in their offices.

Based on quantum physics, this machine is referred to by Dr. Steven Small, MD, of California as "the best diagnostic tool there is." To be clear, only an MD or licensed professional can say such a thing. I am just a biofeedback tech, so I can't say it out loud legally. Dr. Small has been called "doctor of the stars." He said the first thing he does with a new patient is to put them on the SCIO when I saw him speak in Budapest.

You will not find a lot of information on biofeedback online, as the government and others are against its success. By law, we can only treat stress and provide relaxation using this technique. Luckily, all the things that create stress show up in the many programs on this machine, so I always learn the truth, and can share it with professionals of my clients. I have shared same with many professionals over fourteen years.

There are different makers of biofeedback machines, and based on my years of experience, you get what you pay for. But mine (and Eductor), due to the brilliance of their inventor, are more than just biofeedback machines. Nelson designed the QXCI as the first model because he had an autistic child he wanted to help by creating a medical device. The intelligence in my machine leaves nearly all of western medicine in the dust because it is not linear, and the truth is not either—quantum physics proves that the truth is holographic, remember.

When I purchased my EPFX/SCIO from Canada, it came with a long reading list of books on quantum physics so we could understand it. I especially remember Lynn McTaggart's *The Field*, *The Holographic Universe* by Michael Talbot, and Valerie Hunt's *The Infinite Mind*. I felt like a kid in a candy store, experiencing one great idea after another, moments that I'll never forget. I thought of my inventor father and smiled, as I finally found the real truth after years of searching for it in Philosophy, Semantics, etc. after taking hundreds of classes and reading even more books. I felt it in my gut; I knew it was one hundred percent true and that there was such a thing now as the real truth. I smiled from ear to ear with enormous happiness and restored faith and hope.

The reality was that I was so sick and weak in Las Vegas at that time, trying to manage twenty-eight furnished apartment units in a changing neighborhood so full of crime that they called it " naked city." I went to a wellness clinic some holistic healers had just started and received QXCI treatments by a smart practitioner from Naples, Florida. Right off, I was amazed at the hundreds of programs. The treatments this lady gave me really helped, and when she told me there was a new, upgraded machine coming out, I had to come up with money I didn't have to order it. When it arrived from Canada, I got a laptop for it, but both it and the machine stayed on the floor for two months because I was too sick and weak to do anything but walk around them.

I knew I would die if I didn't get to Santa Monica, California, where the week of Beginners training on the machine would begin.

So, I got a sitter for my two dogs, and it was a slow, step-by-step process to get me to the airport, through security, into LAX, and to the training center. There I met Nirvana, an incredible teacher, and I told her how ill I was and how I hoped I could do the week. She set me up with another EPFX/SCIO tech that afternoon. The tech sat at her desk with her laptop open and her EPFX/SCIO on as I spent an hour telling her about my illness. She kept clicking away on the machine's programs, and when she said we were done, I felt like we had just started. I wandered back to my hotel and fell onto the bed, dead exhausted.

That is, until I woke up to go to the bathroom again—and again—as the veritable s—t hit the fan. I never realized one body could hold so much waste until the morning, when I had my last trip to the toilet. She sure cleaned my clock with that one-hour treatment, because I felt so much better. I couldn't wait to eat breakfast and go to class. After one week there, I got my life back, learning how to use the biofeedback machine called the EPFX/SCIO. The irony was that the inventor inventing it didn't mean he knew yet how to USE it, so it was us in the class having to take hints to learn that ourselves.

Later, I returned to Santa Monica for the Advanced class, and then I went to Puerto Vallarta for a week and then to Budapest, Hungary, where the inventor now lives as Desiré Dubounet, female, proudly transgender, born with male and female genitalia. This is a very complicated machine, and most owners are from Europe, Canada, and the United States. Because my machine diagnosed me correctly when a lifetime of seeing MDs couldn't, I was able to treat myself on it weekly and scramble the frequencies of pathogens, feed myself healthy depleted nutrients, teach myself what it knew, and turn my health around. Yes, since I'd had Lyme disease and its nasty coinfections for over fifty years, it took time, but each month was better than the last, and I felt the positives, used my truth tools, and read my truth heroes. I went to seminars, took classes, read the *Townsend Letter for Doctors and Patients*.

I also learned of a few genetic flaws I had that interfered with my recovery before this, as they had to do with reduced immunity. The SCIO frequencies were all determined over ten years by the Inventor Nelson, including these genetic flaws. The EPFX/SCIO has all the Rife frequencies, Chinese medicine, all the Standard Process supplement frequencies, GUNA, electroacupuncture, polarity, chromosomes, detoxification, miasms, pH, volts, amps and resistance, cellular vitality, EEG, EKG, pathogens, organs, Seyle graphs of energy phases, tissue salts, blood, toxic damp heat, radiation, positive and negative, mitochondria, solvents, phenols, parasites, RNA/DNA, Candida, ESP, brain tumors, cancer, emotional issues, vaccines, blockages, grounding, aura protection, endothelium aging, aberrant signals, organs, arterial blockage, metabolism issues, cerebral ischemia, encephalitis, solar radiation, food poisoning (can last twelve years if not treated), aneurisms, degeneration wave forms, hypertension, dental caries, malnutrition, autism, bipolar disorder, depression, cellular nuclear injury, Geopathic Stressors, heart bundle branch block, alopecia, immune transfer factors, and on and on. You can see how sophisticated this machine is. Professor Nelson identifies each frequency himself and is constantly updating new ones. Updated programs are available to run right along with existing programs and improve their abilities for owners of the SCIO and Eductor on a regular basis as the Inventor finds new improvements.

I should add that the private company that distributed my EPFX/SCIO is no longer in business, and EPFX/SCIOs hit the market discounted. Some training on the machine is also available online, so I think it's a great deal if you have the head for it. Also, as already mentioned, the latest upgrade, the Eductor, is available at www.

qxsubspace.com, and www.whitedovehealing.com, and I think all professionals should have one or the other. The inventor has nothing to do with selling his inventions.

6. Syncrometer

The brilliant microbiologist Hulda Regehr Clark, PhD, ND, designed this testing device herself so that patients would be able to test themselves and verify the research she discusses in her six fantastic books. She used her Syncrometer to write *The Cure for All Diseases* (cancers, advanced cancers, HIV/AIDS, etc.) first and it is now translated into twelve languages. I will discuss her six great books in the second chapter.

The beauty of this invention is that you can make your own Syncrometer from scratch. Her books discuss its use, and a manual is available with directions (www.syncrometer.com). The www.drclarkstore.com (866-372-5275) is run by her family at the Self Health Resource Center, where her SyncroZap, Ozonators, her famous "zappers," supplements, and parts are all available. The Syncrometer is about the size of a shoebox, and Syncrometer Science offers a lab manual for $25. and the *Syncrometer Basics* DVD for $20. Her kids are wonderful to work with and can answer all your questions. The cost of putting the Syncrometer together should be about $150. You can verify everything she says using this machine, and learn to test your body for everything for a lot less than the biofeedback machines.

We have now concluded the first chapter and our introduction to the best truth tools I know of in the world. You have seen the overlap of the first four categories—all use kinesiology/Dowsing. All are energy testers. The last two use electrical current energy testers. These tools are simple to use and to learn about, and for the enormous benefits they give us, they are real fun and informative new life savers. Having all of these tools is not necessary, by any means; you can start with the first two. Remember, this path took me several years, and you may not need much. With my case, a very complicated one, you can see how many dimensions an illness can take via my experience and tools. Even if your condition is as complex as mine, you have a huge shortcut to identifying what you need by using the tools I found and get big help fast for relief and recovery. It's a win-win situation no matter what your illness is, small, large, severe, slight, acute, chronic, lifelong or recent. I got my hope back and so will you.

CHAPTER 2

Truth Heroes and Their Books

———

In this chapter, I discuss over twenty-five authors whose books were instrumental to my success in overcoming the effects of a complicated, devastating illness. Of the hundreds of other books I read in order to recover, these were the cream on top. I'll give a description of each so that you can choose which you think you'd benefit from the most. A number appearing after the book's title indicates what I calibrated it on the Map of Consciousness. All of these are over 700, a very high level of truth and consciousness.

1. David R. Hawkins, MD, PhD

I've already introduced you to this spiritual genius and to *Power vs. Force: The Hidden Determinants of Human Behavior* (885), which I referred to as the most important book I ever read. I was enchanted by Dr. Hawkins's perspective when I went to his lectures in Sedona. Thank God he had a great sense of humor to break the trance of concentration I was in. I subscribed to his DVDs of the lectures and read most of his books, and if you contact www.veritaspub.com for a catalog you will find many DVDs to choose from in order to hear this great man yourself. There are also study groups that discuss his work.

Dr. Hawkins discusses power in sports, the arts, physical health, and religion. Even words like *aesthetic* can be positive and enlivening whereas *artsy* can be negative and weakening; *confident* is positive; *arrogant* is weakening; *holistic* is positive, but *analytic* is weakening, and so on. The book contains two entire pages of these word patterns. I think I felt as if I'd been unconscious my whole life before reading *Power vs. Force* because I didn't see the big picture or the new paradigm. After I read it, I changed my perception and perspective completely. By raising my own level of consciousness, I could raise that of many others. Dr. Hawkins's chart shows how one individual at level 500 on the Map of Consciousness counterbalances 750,000 people below level 200, which is all negative and false. Be sure to get a copy of the Map of Consciousness to use as a guide toward your recovery by calibrating your choices, information, doctors, tests, beliefs—you name it. This is the most empowering tool you will ever find, and the more you use it, the more it will allow you to stay high on the truth plane.

2. Hulda Regehr Clark, PhD, ND

I've already introduced you to this great German microbiologist who spent her entire life doing remarkable research to find the truth about the causes of disease. Her six books are *The Cure for All Diseases*, *The Cure for All Cancers*, *The Cure for All Advanced Cancers*, *The Cure for HIV/AIDS*, *The Prevention of All Cancers*, and her last one, *The Prevention and Cure for All Cancers*. I calibrate 930 on *The Cure for All Cancers*, and anyone who has cancer issues should read her books for the truths about cancer. It shows you how fast you can cure it—in a matter of weeks—and how to build your health after that and avoid its causes in the future.

Dr. Clark offers so many cases and mentions things like water softeners and Clorox in the water supply (I never use this toxic product), and each book will show you other things. Her discussion of solvents such as isopropyl alcohol, benzene, and so on that are used in shampoos, cosmetics, and packaging are major contributors, especially combined with particular parasites, in creating cancers. Using my biofeedback machine, I have seen a great many clients who have parasite problems and don't know it. I again saw the truth in this as I reread Dr. Clark's great books recently (taking hydrochloric acid (Hcl) with meals for digestion and keep parasites at bay, for instance).

Remarkably, Dr. Clark also tells us how to clean out each of these causes and very specifically kill the parasites in question. I remember when I first read Dr. Clark's books after they came out, I used her advice about cleaning out my house of toxic chemicals, the garage, and so on. Some people feel she is very demanding, but remember— she is talking about cures, not treatments, of very difficult illnesses. You can choose what you need to follow. It takes work to heal, and it takes energy.

Dr. Clark's research should be taught in medical schools worldwide, but it won't surprise you that they have tried to suppress her great work, as the money stream for cancer clinics and drugs and so on would run dry. If you have any serious illness—or want to prevent them—her books are must-reads. www.newcenturypress.com also has her books, as does Amazon, but the www.drclarkstore.com is family run and can answer any questions. They have zappers and much more.

In *The Cure for All Diseases*, Dr. Clark says, "All illness comes from two causes: parasites and pollutants." I have read that parasites cause eighty percent of all illnesses, and Americans think we don't get parasites. Wrong. The TV program *Monsters Inside Me* is bringing to light the damage parasites do and how slow doctors are to recognize them. I see the damage to patients waiting weeks for test results that my biofeedback machine could identify in an hour.

Another thing Dr. Clark says is that "there is no disease that can outwit you if you know enough about it." She says you need to boil milk for ten seconds before drinking it because salmonella and shingella are not killed by pasteurization and homogenization. Those two culprits kept showing up in me on my own tests, and I kept wondering where they were coming from. I'd forgotten that she recommended boiling dairy until I reread her books, and now I do that little ritual with the grass-fed milk available now, when I bring it home with a smile. Knowledge is the truth that sets you free.

I can't tell you how many tips are in each of Hulda's books—things like the fact that quelling alcoholism needs ergot (mold) and beryllium detoxification, not just avoidance. Also, the presence of isopropyl alcohol is found in one hundred percent of cancer patients, benzene in one hundred percent of HIV/AIDS patients, wood alcohol (natural in orange juice) in one hundred percent of diabetes patients, and xylene and toluene in one hundred percent of Alzheimer's patients. She lists products that contain these solvents. My EPFX/SCIO lists solvents I find in myself, and I play Medical Detective, trying to find out where I got them, the way I do if I see GMO food and other bad boys. Hulda was an unsung truth hero who still deserves a Nobel Prize. Between her Syncrometer device and her books, you can build a very strong health army.

3. Ryke Geerd Hamer, MD

This remarkable doctor found German New Medicine after his son was shot dead in Munich. His wife died from the grief of that loss, and he himself got testicular cancer. He saw that there had to be an emotional component to illness. At that time, he was head internist at Munich University's oncology center, so he asked each of his patients if they'd had any emotional event preceding the onset of their cancer. All of them said yes. That was the beginning of Dr. Hamer's research into biological conflict as cause of illness. Because his books are in German, the best information on the German New Medicine is online and definitely worth your printing out several pages, including an interview with him. I found the book *Biogenealogy: Decoding the Psychic Roots of Illness: Freedom from the Ancestral Origins of Disease* by Patrick Obissier a very good source of information on Hamer's years of research and highly recommend it. Dr. Hamer proved that all illnesses, from colds to cancer, are caused by "unexpected, unresolved shock."

When I first read this, I recalled an incident when I was eight years old. The kid next door hit me in the head with an axe. All I saw was blood, and I ran home. I assume somebody brought me to the hospital, but I don't remember anything other than seeing blood all over me. Unexpected? For sure. I realized that over the many years since, I or others had always been hitting me at that spot on my head or that things had hit me near that very site. I saw a pattern over the years, but when I read this book—bingo. That old injury had created an energy pattern that kept repeating the negative injury attractor, and it was never "resolved." I removed it with the pendulum spin left, and added back love energy to fill the space I created by the removal.

To really point this out, as I was reading this very book, and I put it down to get something out of the bottom of a box in the kitchen. I had just moved and hadn't unpacked everything yet. I was feeling around for the skewers at the bottom, and when I felt them with my fingers, I pulled to get them out of the bottom. But I yanked them too hard, stabbing myself at the top of my nose, right near that same spot. Blood was everywhere again, and I was so mad at myself for proving this point one hundred percent just as I was reading the book. Dummy! Well, Dr. Hamer's "Hamer Herd" in the brain is known worldwide now, and it's on my machine under the brain scan, showing emotional components leading toward cancer. Stress molecules are so strong they can kill you, but your brain keeps them from doing that. After the CAT scan was invented, Hamer was able to show where in the brain the event was stored and, further, could tell where in the body illness would manifest later if the trauma was not resolved. I cleared myself of the axe event right after my last self-injury, needless to say.

Dr. Hamer shows how these conflicts can be passed down genetically from generation to generation. I spent a lot of time thinking about my childhood after that and clearing unresolved issues there first before dealing with those from my adulthood. Talk about the "baggage" that we carry—who knew? When we clear these using Dowsing, the pendulum, or the Yuen Method, we clear them for future generations, too. So I got busy.

Sadly, I can't find information on where Dr. Hamer is now. Germany went after Dr. Hamer and took his license away since all the income-producing linear drugs and treatments had no place in this new truth picture. I read that they went after him from France and jailed him in Spain. If he is still alive, he would be in his eighties now. But German New Medicine, which has a cancer cure rate of 92 percent, survives, and more and more is filtering in globally. He has the iron rule for cancer. This is a must-read. German New Medicine is here to stay. Thank you Dr. Hamer.

4. Kam Yuen, DC

You have already met Dr. Yuen in chapter one, so I won't say much more here because his writings are all about www.yuenmethod.com, which I already described as a very important truth tool for health, power, and freedom on all levels using his level one, two, and three workbooks, available on Amazon.com also.

5. Professor Bill Nelson/Desiré Dubounet

I have also previously mentioned in detail this inventor of the EPFX/SCIO (and its current upgrade, the Eductor). Instead of writings, he "wrote" his knowledge and developments into the base computer programs for the machine. Another genius. The Eductor is his upgrade of the EPFX/SCIO.

6. William B. Ferril, MD

During the ten years I spent in bed suffering with chronic fatigue, I read the *Townsend Letter for Doctors & Patients* voraciously for answers and found an interesting article by Dr. Ferril about hormones. I called his office in Whitefish, Montana, and learned of his terrific book *The Body Heals*. After being graduated from medical school, Dr. Ferril wasn't finding the information he learned in school to be working for him in practice. He sold his farm and took five years to investigate the truth via many research studies over many years. *The Body Heals* shows how to heal so many things "without drugs or medical procedures." This great doctor wrote over six hundred pages of breakthrough information you won't find anywhere else, and it really helped me use his discoveries in my health project. For example, here is his take on "the Seven Paths to an Old Body":

   a) The give and take of hormones
   b) The rusting process
   c) The hardening process

d) Low-cell-voltage syndrome
e) Deficient or excessive molecular building parts
f) Failure to take out the cellular trash
g) A preponderance of energies that maim compared to the energies that heal

Dr. Ferril clears up the mistakes made by other doctors and sets the truth free. His book *Glandular Failure-Caused Obesity* is another truth teller. His books and articles are available at www.thebodyheals.com (406-863-9906). By the way, when Dr. Atkins (the Cardiologist MD of Atkins Diet fame) passed away, Dr. Ferril was asked to take over the Atkins newsletter, which he did, although he had to eventually give it up due to lack of time. He is truly an original thinker, and through him I discovered I was gluten intolerant, which made a huge difference in my health when I quit it, among other things.

7. Richard Horowitz, MD

The inimitable Dr. Horowitz has been a champion of Lymees and chronic illness for decades. When his book *Why Can't I Get Better? Solving the Mystery of Lyme and Chronic Disease* finally was announced, I preordered it, afraid it would sell out before I could get one. His next book will be out January 2017, so you might want to preorder it too.

There could not be a more thorough and complete professional analysis of chronic illnesses than this huge book, which compiles every level of expertise and the experience of Dr. Horowitz himself over his many years in practice in Hyde Park, New York. He has survived great personal and professional attacks. God bless this great truth hero. This book can be read by doctors and patients alike as it addresses Lyme and chronic illness on all fronts. I felt wonderful after I read it because when I realized I had Lyme, almost no information about it was out there. I took bits from the *Townsend* and Dr. Klinghardt's website and made choices by the seat of my pants long before this book came out. Luckily, I saw that I had done everything recommended in the book for Lyme. Big exhale there.

This is a book written for professionals and may overwhelm the lay Lymee, so be advised. In this tome, the only other book Dr. Horowitz recommended was *Journey* by Brandon Bays, which I ordered right away, since it investigated the emotional component patients need to address. I will talk about Brandon Bays later, as her work is so valuable. She is surely most evolved in dealing with emotional hidden elements that cause illness.

8. Russell M. Blaylock, MD

I found *Health and Nutrition Secrets That Can Save Your Life: Harness Your Body's Natural Healing Powers* by Dr. Blaylock after I read a review and bought another of his books, *Excitotoxins: The Taste That Kills*, which was a huge eye-opener about MSG and other dangers.

But *Health and Nutrition Secrets* was the "mother lode" for sure for truth news you can use. Dr. Blaylock's many years as a cardiac surgeon taught him so much that other MDs simply didn't know. In his introduction, Dr. Blaylock says: "Trauma to the body—even to the head alone—greatly increases the body's metabolic rate. In fact, the metabolic rates of many trauma patients resemble those of long-distance runners...such stresses to the body cause a very rapid depletion of water-soluble vitamins and many minerals."

I had an auto accident in 1973 and suffered a head injury. My biofeedback machine always shows me as deficient in B vitamins, vitamin C, and major minerals, and I could only imagine how all my freeloading pathogens were eating them until I read this. Despite all the supplements I take, I still have difficulty holding on to my minerals and vitamin B. It's the head-injury trauma, Pyroluria, and stress. I found lots of news I could use in this book, and you will too.

With each of these truth heroes, I found answers and took another rung up the truth ladder toward health and more energy for healing. I keep these essential books in my library for further research, and they make my foundation grow and expand—along with my self-confidence and faith in my future.

Dr. Blaylock has a ton of information in this book about pre- and post operation advice that is a must-read if you're a surgical candidate, like it's "vital to take 2000 mg of methyl cobalamin (best B12 form) daily for at least a month before surgery." He talks about all the flaws in the way protocol for surgical patients is done now, which will surprise you. He also provides extensive information about heart issues like atherosclerosis, strokes, heart failure, cardiovascular disease and natural treatments. Lots of "yes!" moments in this great read by a doctor who tells it like it is.

9. Joan Matthews Larson, PhD

I found Joan Matthews Larson's book 7 *Weeks to Emotional Healing*, now out of print, years ago, before I knew I had a physical illness, when I thought my problems were "all in my head," like the allopathic MDs told me. This book leaped into my hand at a bookstore, and its first chapter was entitled *"It's Not All in Your Mind."*

Really? I saw a list of "biotypes of emotions" that led to the charts that indicated which chapters you should read accordingly. There was one about fatigue, one on depression, low blood sugar, anxiety, irritability/anger/violence, high histamine (manic), low thyroid, Candida/food allergies/memory, and chemical sensitivities. Larson talks about genetic history and "how nutrient deprivation cripples us emotionally." Her book *Seven Weeks to Sobriety* is still available, as is her book *Depression-Free Naturally*, which has most of the same information. This is how I learned about Candida and Pyroluria, and when I tested for them, I found I had high scores in both. Like Larson said under "Pyroluria as a Cause of Anxiety," the loss of vitamin B6 and zinc it causes is a "psychiatric disaster." This was big news I could use, and I will discuss Pyroluria later because it is a mostly unknown but very serious kidney molecule that doubles under stress in those of us who suffer anxiety and tension. It's a nerve poison we inherit.

Joan has run the famous Health Recovery Center in Minneapolis for years based on nutritional treatment of addictions, and she worked with Abram Hoffer, MD, the Canadian psychiatrist, and Carl Pfeiffer, MD, of Princeton, who simultaneously discovered the "mauve" factor, or kryptopyrroles, as they studied Schizophrenia. Hoffer cofounded molecular biology with using vitamin B3 to cure Schizophrenia. That was when all the psychiatric hospitals emptied as I recall it. Joan is a true champion for her work of identifying the truth about addictions and bad chemistry. God bless this great lady, who is now in her eighties.

10. David Perlmutter, MD

Dr. Perlmutter wrote *Grain Brain: The Surprising Truth about Wheat, Carbs, and Sugar—Your Brain's Silent Killers* fairly recently. It's so chock-full of health-truth news that you won't want to put it down. Dr. Perlmutter is a founding member and fellow of the American Board of Integrative and Holistic Medicine, a neurologist, and a true expert on what we eat and how our brains function. Food is a powerful epigenetic modulator that can change our very DNA. Most of us know about gluten sensitivity and think it affects other people. Alas, it affects most of us. I have Celiac disease, which came from it, and I hope to avoid Alzheimer's disease by banishing gluten. Among the many signs of gluten sensitivity the good doctor lists are "ADHD, ALS, alcoholism, anxiety, Autism, ataxia (loss of balance), autoimmune diseases (diabetes, Hashimoto's thyroiditis, rheumatoid arthritis, etc.)"—and these are just the ones under "A." What's more, this book has a mountain of nutritional information and plans of action on how to help. *Brain Maker: The Power of Gut Microbes to Heal and Protect Your Brain—for Life* is Dr. Perlmutter's latest book, which continues with the most recent studies and information we need to know. Here is his list of the things a C-section can lead to:

* Five times greater risk of allergies
* Three times greater risk of ADHD
* Two times greater risk of autism
* Eighty percent increased risk of Celiac disease
* Fifty percent increased risk of becoming obese as an adult (which connects with dementia later)
* Seventy percent increased risk of type-1 diabetes

A nice young man with a pregnant wife was telling me they'd had to schedule his wife's labor appointment on the hour at the local hospital and that it had to take place during the scheduled time or they would give her a C-section. He told me they said that was common practice now, and I verified this with other friends all over the country. This should be illegal.

Knowledge is power here, and you will realize how to take back your power by reading these books and finding the truth about how our bodies work, how to take control of your health instead of being a victim of the powers that be. You will start to actually feel the difference using these truth tools and reading these books.

11. William Davis, MD

Dr. Davis's specialty is preventive cardiology, and his great book *Wheat Belly: Lose the Wheat, Lose the Weight, and Find Your Path Back to Health* is another pathfinder of truth. I expected this book to repeat the same messages from Dr. Perlmutter's books, but surprisingly it was all new information throughout, although the two books show how the genomes of wheat DNA have been altered on us over the years and all the problems that have now resulted. Dr. Davis has a great sense of humor when describing his findings, making his truths entertaining as well as important.

12. Dietrich Klinghardt, MD

I heard about Dr. Klinghardt through practitioners who studied with him, and their treatments were very helpful to me. I found Dr. Klinghardt's website (www.klinghardtneurobiology.com) and printed out articles galore on Lyme disease (which he had himself and is a top expert on) and autism in children born to Lyme parents.

Since Dr. Klinghardt is German born, he doesn't write in English, but he has a very busy practice in Kirkland, Washington, where the most difficult cases find him. I've seen Dr. Klinghardt at Lyme seminars, and he is a genius, devoted to sharing his knowledge with patients and professionals alike. Later I will discuss Pyroluria, common in Lymees, as well as Autism, and I consider Dr. Klinghardt the top expert today. He has a one-hour YouTube talk on Pyroluria that in my opinion is more informative than any other source. He tells in detail the story of this unrecognized condition I learned about first through Joan Matthews Larson, but his research on this and everything else he studies is top-notch. Since MDs in Germany also learn natural cures, Dr. Klinghardt has had a much more holistic education. He's a truly devoted scientist, and the Lyme information I found on his website when there was so little on Lyme anywhere before now was key to my being able to help myself. His students love what they learn—the ART testing especially. He believes that microorganisms like Lyme feel our huge electro-smog increase, plus microwaves and satellites, and react as if they are being attacked by reproducing at any cost. He was the first to say this, and I think he's right on the money.

13. Stephen Harrod Buhner

This super master herbalist also heads the GAIA Institute. At first, I found a slim book that he wrote—*Healing Lyme*—and its simplicity and herbal treatments were very appealing for such a complex disease. I recommended it to people who discovered they had Lyme disease so that they wouldn't be terrified and do something rash! (There's good news, and there's bad news—and then there's double bad news. Lyme is the latter.)

When his second book, *Healing Lyme Disease Coinfections: Complementary and Holistic Treatments for Bartonella and Mycoplasma*, came out, it was twice as thick as his first book, and I wondered why—especially because I have these two coinfections. Well, they deserved the space. When I finished this book (I only scanned some of the herb details that were over my head), I had an all-new perspective of this Lyme and coinfections picture. Stephen has a mind like a steel trap about his research, and when I put the book down, I just sat there, realizing that he showed how these little microorganisms have been evolving over billions of years and that we sort of just got here, so we couldn't really win this one. He put forth that we each had to become our own doctors, because illnesses today are so much more complex and that no doctor could keep up with all the multiple symptoms in the future. Having these two coinfections of Lyme can be worse than the Lyme itself. I can attest to that.

Stephen Buhner has spent so much time since the original *Healing Lyme* book writing about it that his second edition of the original book with all its updates was twice as big, plus, he wrote another: *Natural Treatments for Lyme Coinfections: Anaplasma, Babesia, and Ehrlichia*. Since I also have Babesia (like Malaria), I had to read it, of course, and I also got *Herbal Antibiotics: Natural Alternatives for Treating Drug-Resistant Bacteria* and *Herbal Antivirals: Natural Remedies for Emerging and Resistant Viral Infections* for my library.

Buhner, this fountain of herbal knowledge, has also written *The Secret Teachings of Plants: The Intelligence of the Heart in the Direct Perception of Nature* (the GAIA Institute's message) and spiritually is totally evolved. The only thing I don't agree with in his works is his skepticism about kinesiology's arm testing. Yes, it can be influenced by emotions, but not if one is clear and centered and using the introduction I talk about, which he doesn't know of—yet!

Stephen Harrod Buhner is a gift to mankind for his numerous books on ecological medicine and plants. His recent efforts to help Lymees by producing all these books for us in quick succession were truly a labor of love, and we Lymees love you back, Stephen. Thank you.

14. Michael J. Lincoln, PhD

I was taking a class for certification in Theta Healing when the teacher held up a book called *Messages from the Body: Their Psychological Meaning (The Body's Desk Reference)* by Michael J. Lincoln, PhD, the condensed version of a huge volume consisting of over seven hundred pages. This volume (as well as Lincoln's other great books) is available only at www.talkinghearts.net and will just knock your socks off when you look up various ailments and the psychological causes in this "dictionary."

Although Dr. Lincoln has more than enough credentials and experience to write on all these issues, when I was reading the beginning, I realized that nobody could know so much about so much. Although he never says it, I believe he channeled the information in all his terrific books. (I get 875 on the Map of Consciousness.) I love books that were channeled, from Sanaya Roman's to Helen Schucman's *A Course in Miracles.* I don't try to explain it; I just appreciate the telepathic gifts of the people who can access brilliant messages like this.

I scanned the entire book page by page and read each of the many items that described some illness I had or that other people close to me had, and it was spot on, one after another and none wrong. Everything revealed was accurate. For example, I had colitis when my husband and I chose to separate years ago, and then I had it again more recently—it had come back. I lost twenty pounds years ago with it, and this is what Lincoln says:

> Self-deprivation. They have a guilty feeling of unlovability and a great need to be loved that is prevented fulfillment by self-punishing self-denial for presumed transgressions that the outside world is unaware of. There is desperation for affection they never got that results in self-denigration and pessimism…
>
> There is a considerable feeling of undue burdens, emotional strain, and loneliness. They are very insecure, and they have a very difficult time letting go of that which is over and done with. It came from over-exacting parents who imposed an experience of intense oppression, over-responsibility, and defeat.

There is more to colitis, but this is the gist of it, and it fits like a glove. Reading all my illness history came up with similar family-origin causation, and I will add Lyme disease here to show you:

Sealed Unit: They are an "urban hermit," an achieve-aholic, and a self-denying performance maniac. They feel that they have to take care of everything because no one else will, or they'll do it all wrong. They are so caught up in taking care of business and running the show that they have real trouble with intimacy, vulnerability, and emotional commitment. Underneath all this, they are support-starved, frustrated, and resentful. It all got started in a "never good enough" parenting situation, in which they were put on a very conditional love basis—they had to perform for their breakfast. However, they never seemed to come up to snuff, so there is a subconscious, subtle, and subterranean self-disgust and lack of self-confidence. What happened is they became hooked to the "tie that grinds" in an engulfed symbiosis with their parent, who in turn functionally relied on them to rescue them...

Now you can see why I had so much therapy. But reading these true descriptions of my truckloads of baggage was incredible, because it just released them one by one. After I finished, I felt like my load was somehow finally gone. Everybody is in this book, so it's like a cleanser that shouldn't be overlooked, an investment in truth telling by a great dedicated healer and seer. Afterward, I bought Lincoln's other books, and they were just as spot on as this one. His book *Allergies and Aversions*, for instance, helped me further refine the causes of my allergies. All professionals in healing should carry these books; they are in a league of their own for understanding truths behind illness.

15. John Harrison, MD
Years ago, I found Dr. Harrison's *Love Your Disease: It's Keeping You Healthy*. The title of this book captivated me early on in my search for

truth. I played amateur psychologist for years with a friend from middle school who was then also an avid searcher for information. Especially after I started the first Adult Children of Alcoholics meeting in Las Vegas through Al-Anon, it was like a game she and I played on the phone, since she lived in New Jersey. We would describe the case and predict what would happen to people through our powers of deduction based on all the psychology books we read. Trying to explain our families, both touched by alcoholism and crazy behavior patterns all our lives, we called it self-therapy. So, this book by Harrison was flying way out of the orb of Psych 101 then, saying things like the following:

> Every disease we give ourselves has advantages. The advantages lie in helping us to maintain a belief system about ourselves, others, and the world, which, although damaging to us in some way, effectively masks more deep-seated and fundamental fears. By becoming ill, we spare ourselves the trauma of examining those aspects of ourselves we have chosen to suppress.

Since I already knew that blaming others was not an option for healing, that only the truth was, I did a lot of thinking as I read this book. It wasn't until many years later that it popped up in my head again, when the worst thing that ever happened to me besides the death of my father when I was twelve occurred. In Las Vegas a bad mayor and bad cop made me tear down my twenty-eight apartments there *and* wanted to charge me $80,000. to do it. I got it done for $20,000 and couldn't fight them for two years, and it left me with an acre of land and no income. I spent a year in bed when that was over, after I found a buyer for the land and moved to Arizona. It was that year in bed followed by nine more years of off-and-on chronic fatigue before I learned about Lyme disease and remembered what Dr. Harrison said.

It was something about the fact that getting sick was a better choice than facing the fear you had, and he was right. I was mentally and emotionally bankrupted by this totally illegal and unfair act of the city against me and others and by being helpless to fight them, which they knew. I just couldn't take any more, and so I got sick, hiding with my two dogs in Arizona, where I didn't know anyone and could watch TV and not think anymore. Later, I started reading again, and there was Dr. Harrison's book from years before, because I save books I believe in.

There are other books you have probably noticed by now that show the real causes of illness that all jive with each other and reaffirm the emotional charges we stack up against ourselves. As I mentioned, they can start prenatally, and they took me years to find. Each factor I discovered, I could release, usually just by reading about it, or if it needed more work, by Dowsing or clearing methods. I feel free as a bird today, free at last, because finding these incredible truth heroes did so much to find me for me and free myself through the discoveries they wanted to share to help others.

It's what they have done for me that make me want to pass the wisdom I learned from them to you. The 1973 book *Primal Man* by Doctors Janov and Holden was the key to all that followed about the primary pain that affects the rest of our lives, creates our personalities, and so on. The only reason I don't list it here is because it's from so far back, but it was the beginning of the truth in psychology.

16. Michael Greenwood, MD, and Peter Nunn, MD

The book *Paradox & Healing: Medicine, Mythology & Transformation* is Canadian and fits the truth hero's common denominators when they say right in the introduction:

As practicing physicians, we have come to believe that the denial of feelings—the irrational part of ourselves—will eventually lead to illness and chronic pain. And further, we have seen how far grappling with our despair and our personal paradoxes can lead to healing...by ignoring the emotions, conventional medicine wastes time, money, and energy trying to find rational explanations for disease when there may be none to find. And the enormous effort sometimes undertaken to make a diagnosis may itself, paradoxically, promote illness.

I loved reading this book. The way these two brilliant holistic doctors saw right through all the medical swamp of allopathic medicine to the truth of energy blocks and qi or chi was so smart. Connected with the mythology of fairy tales and our paternalistic culture, it states that "prevention" medicine "not only does not work, but is expensive and potentially harmful, dragging society into a quagmire of expensive medical testing to create the illusion of better health..." Amen.

They follow with examples of medical follies, saying "we could stop spending millions of dollars on an outmoded health-care system that is bankrupting the nation and start a collective transformational journey..." This is where my book feels we can go now. After we find health using the tools and discovering the real information in books like this one by our truth heroes, our energy will return quickly and our self-confidence even faster, because we have tools to use and calibrate with, to remove and add with, and to restore our faith that no way will we ever need to be powerless victims again.

All our cultural, educational, and religious differences won't amount to a hill of beans when we have the simple, powerful, effortless truth in front of us at all times. So, there is no benefit whatsoever in telling lies if you are on the truth side. Only if you are dishonest and trying to victimize others will you lie. Even the fact that people are on different levels of consciousness doesn't change the eternal truth, which is what can be so hopeful when dealing with countries so far apart ideologically. Truth can be tested; opinion can be trashed in the ego bin.

In their fine book, Greenwood and Nunn talk about "the discoveries of the new physics...assert that both aspects of a paradox can and do coexist; and point out that we see the one we set the experiment up to see—the one we want to see. Everything is whole in itself and at the same time part of an infinite number of other wholenesses."

Lastly, they show that "when illness arises through denial, the desire to eradicate it is really an attempt to permanently 'kill' the denied portion of the self...that struggle against the self is ultimately the nature of illness."

17. Brandon Bays

This soulful author's evolved writings are simple to read yet so deep. They take you inside yourself as she delves inside her own self on the soul level. Her egoless, advanced being processes the events in this search, which led her to her technique using a protocol on the emotional journey and physical journey. Her technique workbook allowed me to find my deepest and darkest pain, pain never discovered through any previous therapy or other methods. I think her "no agendas" style of writing allows us to go everywhere without fear of what we may find. Dr. Horowitz's recommendation of Bays's book *Journey* in his own great book *Why Can't I Get Better?* sent me ordering it before I even finished his. Bays talks about seeing her home in California burn down, and it jarred stuck emotional equivalents in my own life.

I always had abandonment issues, and I thought they arose from the death of my father when I was twelve, but what I found using Bays's workbook proved that to be incorrect. Instead, I saw myself in my crib, alone, shortly after I was born. We lived on a farm in Pennsylvania; Daddy worked in the city and came home on weekends. Mom had to do all the farm chores daily, feeding the chickens and milking the cow. As she minded the farm, she took my older brother, Eddy, with her because he could walk, leaving me alone in the crib essentially for two years, until I could walk. This was the abandonment. Nobody came when I cried, when my diapers were dirty, when I was hungry, or when I needed nurturing. I cried and cried, but nobody came, so I stopped crying. To this day, I don't ask for anything because I don't expect anybody to come. When I saw this truth, I cried passionately and deeply for over an hour and a half, going through the entire tissue box, so I knew I'd hit pay dirt. I couldn't release that until I'd found it, and it is extremely hard to find things that happened pre-verbally. The fact that my mother and I had different O blood types—Rh positive and Rh negative—was also part of my earliest entry to life, so rejection and abandonment were like the wallpaper for me. They were always there.

Brandon Bays's other three books were also very rewarding reads in moving me forward spiritually, like her statement that "creative solutions, conscious answers, inspired ideas, and effulgent abundance all arise from the unobscured awareness that is your own self, and this same boundless self is inviting you to take your lampshade off. Life is calling you to stop playing small; it is beckoning you into greatness." So, off came my lampshade, because as Bays ends: "Consciousness *is* the new currency. In fact, consciousness is the *only* currency that will heal our world." I call her the ethereal pragmatist, and I agree with her whole heartedly.

18. Peter Russell

Reading Russell's *Waking Up in Time: Finding Inner Peace in Times of Accelerating Change* is the only book I found that talks in layman's terms about our acceleration in evolving. In short and succinct chapters, he traces the different ages in our history, like the Industrial Revolution, for example. He shows that with each one, they have speeded up, to where we are now in singularity and a conscious future. Russell received an honors degree in theoretical physics and psychology from the University of Cambridge, where he also studied with Stephen Hawking before earning a master's degree in computer science. After that, it was meditation and Eastern philosophy in India. For East-West balance of course? Then neurophysiology and books like *The Upanishads* and *The Global Brain*. I remember my young niece once asking me if someone's opinion mattered to me. I said, "Only if the person who has an opinion really knows their subject." Well, Russell's opinion in *Waking Up in Time* just got reprinted, so I'm not the only serf who wants his "opinion." Talk about an overview of the destiny of our species that will humble us all. He definitely wins.

19. Louise Hay

This Grand Heroine of self-help, now in her eighties, has given most of us something already. Her book *You Can Heal Your Life* has sold over fifty million copies in several languages. I found her workshops in Las Vegas early on, seeing people like Wayne Dyer and Candice Pert speak there along with the whole roster of spiritual healers she organized. I felt close to Louise Hay, experiencing a tormented childhood, overcoming cervical cancer via alternative methods, being a model and an artist, and authoring many great books available today at www.hayhouse.com. Dubbed "the Queen of the New Age" by the *New York Times*, Louise established the body-mind connection in 1976 with her little blue book, *Heal Your Body*, long before mental causes of physical ailments were even mentioned. I'm sure the enormous gratitude we feel for Louise's help drives her to do more and more as she sees how much it has changed negatives to positives for so many, including me. The spiritual workshops she created introduced me to people I'd never heard of before then and opened my mind 360 degrees after hearing them. God bless you, Louise.

20. Dr. Masaru Emoto

When this Japanese genius came out with his *Messages in Water* series, I couldn't wait to get the latest one, fascinated as the various scientific principles were proven with simple photographs of crystals in water responding to words, music, nature, man-made additives, geography, and so on. The more Dr. Emoto expanded his research, the more his thinking followed it, and *The True Power of Water: Healing and Discovering Ourselves* (Hado) is a tiny tome that simplifies quantum physics principles and discusses Hado medicine. Hado measures vibrations of the body at a cellular level, showing the Hado relations between emotions and parts of the body. In *The Healing Power of Water*, he provides more "information," but each of these eight books is a treasure chest of pictures that truly are worth a thousand words. I've always been amazed at how little we know about water—so essential to life, yet it carved out the Grand Canyon. (*The Mysteries of Water* DVD or on YouTube is a must-see.) Young people can get big input seeing this relationship of water to the environment at an early age using Dr. Emoto's photos. Water is always positive. Say thank you to it, and it will have a positive effect on you—putting "thank you" and "love" and "gratitude" under your glass of water changes the crystals positively. I still do it!

Dr. Emoto placed rice in three separate beakers. The first had "thank you" written on it, and it emitted a strong, pleasant aroma. The second said, "You're an idiot," and that turned the rice black. The third beaker was ignored, and the rice rotted. He stated that this should show us how to treat children, since indifference causes the greatest harm. Hatred, rage, and annoyance give feedback, so the negative thinker pollutes his own body's water.

21. Hal Huggins, former DDS

It's All in Your Head by Hal Huggins was the first book recommended to me at my first holistic health fair that changed my sick life, because it blew the whistle on mercury amalgam silver fillings that were making us sick. The American Dental Association won't admit it to this day. His second book, *Uninformed Consent*, was another important revealing truth teller. Hal Huggins lost his DDS license, as will any dentist who talks about mercury today. In other countries, using amalgam fillings at all is illegal, or a maximum of only four per adult is permitted. Hal Huggins also got MS from all the mercury he inhaled using this super toxic material, as did many other dentists, who also have high suicide rates. Today, dentists have pretty much stopped using mercury, but since a lot of people are having these toxic fillings removed, it is important to find "mercury-free dentists" who know the proper way to remove these fillings by testing to find the highest electrical quadrant and to remove them in the right sequence. If you let an ordinary dentist just take them out any old way (and from the many stories I've heard, this is common practice), you can become very ill. Other good books on the dangers of root canals and such have become available because Hal Huggins had the courage to lead the way.

After reading his books, I tested for mercury and as I mentioned, had the highest numerical score of sixty-five, that the Nevada clinic ever saw. It was supposed to be below three. Astonishing. I called Tom Levy, MD, and he also said to get the dental work done ASAP with that score. Then my dental revisions began. I realized that my depression, so severe sometimes that it paralyzed me, was from all that toxic mercury, because since I had it removed, I've never been depressed again. Mold and dental-work story coming later.

22. Stuart Wilde

You remember the line from *Star Wars*: "Let the Force be with you"? Well, *The Force* by Stuart Wilde had to be its origin, because this thin little seventy-five pages says it all. Your higher self, or that energy body, the living light, what have you, is finding uncluttered purity inside you as the force that wants you to carry its light.

While I was going through so much pain and suffering, being down on myself and forlorn, I only had my books—and they were all about illness. Finding the upbeat, hilarious, brilliant work of Stuart Wilde was a godsend. His truths supported my life, my being, my light, with the simplest, most profound lessons ever. The son of a British diplomat, he had a worldliness that only grew as he traveled around the world so many times in his quest for knowledge. So, he got the big picture down right in all his books, and *The Force* was my lantern of light. His *Infinite Self: 33 Steps to Reclaiming Your Inner Power* also helped me understand things and shore up the self-esteem that was leaking out of me daily from the stress of being ill. He pulled me back to the truths and out of the "poor me's" because he talked on the truth-and-nothing-but-the-truth plane only, and it feels good there.

The truth always feels good, because even if the news isn't good, you can change that if you deal with it truthfully. Lies and denial and layers of cover-ups make a house of cards that lead to illness and unhappiness. Wilde opens the *Infinite Self* by saying, "The *33 Energies of Man* was an ancient teaching...from the Taoists in China...said to flow from a higher plane into the earth dimension—a bit like a freeway built of light—to allow humans an exit out of the emotions and thought forms of this evolution into a higher consciousness."

So, instead of thinking about where it hurts, I thought about what lessons God was giving me through this experience. I have felt many times that I was learning everything about health cures because I was destined to use this knowledge later somehow, and voilà, I'm writing this book now to share it with you. I realize I need to stay on the higher plane to be happy, sick or well, because it's staying with the truth that sets me free, makes me feel good, and sees my higher self and not my lower, lead me. Because this force is in me, I love myself. Wilde puts the power back inside the individual you, and nobody does it better.

23. Amit Goswami, PhD

For those who saw the movie *What the Bleep Do We Know?* that took the world by storm some time ago with its clever production and a lot of brilliant speakers interjected throughout, you'll remember Amit Goswami, Professor Emeritus of physics at the Institute of Theoretical Sciences at the University of Oregon. That movie moved me to the core because I didn't know squat about quantum physics or quantum mechanics then, and this film almost scared me with its introduction to it in such a humorous story. I saw it five times before I bought a copy, and then I watched it ten more times and wasn't scared anymore.

In *The Self-Aware Universe: How Consciousness Creates the Material World*, Goswami explains in layman's terms the synthesis of spirituality and science in such beautiful prose. I loved his *Physics of the Soul* and *The Visionary Window* as well. Goswami is the perfect perception wand of learning because he is the best of both worlds: spiritual roots from his birthplace of India and science from spending his adult life in the West. He has a truly unique perspective on the big picture. Well, in his case, the even-bigger-than-that picture.

I calibrated Goswami's book *The Visionary Window* at 995, the highest of any I tested, tied with Dr. Emoto's *The True Power of Water: Healing and Discovering Ourselves*. His *Physics of the Soul* is at 970, so what more can one say about him? Except maybe that we hope he leaves his brain to the Smithsonian.

I never felt that he lost me in his easy explanations of some complex ideas, as if he were the compassionate author who never made you feel lost despite his genius as a contemporary thinker and expert on consciousness. I get so excited reading Goswami's explanations. Of course, don't quiz me on it later because, like quantum physics, I can't explain it even to my dog, but I go along for the thrill of the ride. Reading about his thinking is akin to listening to great music in its expansiveness and lack of linear faults of Western education.

24. Ken Wilber

Although Ken Wilber is known in intellectual circles, the new edition of his book *Up from Eden: A Transpersonal View of Human Evolution* was a great read. You have noticed my penchant for human evolution and consciousness, and Wilber does such a magnificent job explaining the stages of our evolution from being unconscious to consciousness in stages of transcendence. This is pretty deep reading but very worthwhile about the Atman project and more.

I would love to mention other great authors and books, but essentially these were the most helpful to me in my search for truth to bring me back my health and take back my power. All are over 700 on the Map of Consciousness; some are as high as 995. I was going to list their calibrations but then decided it would be better to provide a description and allow you to determine what resonates with you. You can calibrate those that attract you the most. The following are other resources besides individual authors that may pique your interest.

25. *Life Extension* Magazine and Its Medical Advisory Board

This is a remarkable monthly that does its own research on key topics connected with aging. Some of the best holistic MDs and PhDs sit on its medical advisory board, and for a very modest membership fee, you get really cutting-edge information about natural healing. What's more, they produce the products that are useful for their discoveries, and I have found no solvents in any of them. (I found a lot of others had benzene, isopropyl alcohol, or the residue of other solvents used in cleaning the capsules, as required by law.) Their extensive product list is reasonable, and I have liked all the ones I've used very much. It's really like one-stop shopping—plus they offer blood-testing panels for many things. They do truly independent research.

Life Extension's articles are great. I had Sinusitis for years. Its article "Fungal Infections and Sinus Problems" was spot on. More news I could use. They discuss the health-care crisis, anxiety, mood disorders, and everything else. I really look forward to receiving their new issues for the latest information. They say:

> Speak up...before an illness bankrupts you. Only the Life Extension Foundation dares to challenge the FDA's

incompetent and corrupt prescription-drug approval process…will send you free information about highly effective
medicines not approved by the FDA but legally available to
Americans. There are now thousands of useful medical ther-
apies available in Europe and other parts of the world that the
FDA is keeping from you.

I have found this to be true, and they have the facts—like the 5,300
percent increase in the price of Doxycycline, which I used to take
for Lyme. I also like that they take political stands to clean up this
health-care mess and really help people the way doctors should.
(800-678-8989 or www.LifeExtension.com.)

26. Tony Hsieh

I loved reading *Delivering Happiness: A Path to Profits, Passion, and
Purpose*, a delightful tale about Tony Hsieh's success story in a flash.
As the CEO of Zappos.com when he wrote this, he starts with how
his first business adventure as a child was a worm farm. His Asian
parents were very supportive, and he always left the door open as he
made and kept friendships and connections and went through all the
pitfalls common to small businesses. At one point, he and the employees all had to live together in one apartment to save costs.

Where it gets great is when he got his first offer to buy his business, an offer of over $1 million, and after a lot of soul searching,
Tony realized for the first time that it wasn't about money. He turned
it down. The Zappos "culture" he then created is well known today
and is being adopted by multiple giant corporations who used to
treat customers like numbers and employees no better. The Zappos
culture makes the employees as well as the customers happy by
making efficiency and ideas the main attractions, ensuring two-day

deliveries from a giant delivery center in Kentucky. Tony also retained a lot of bonding with the buddies he started with. Everyone knows that Amazon bought him out for over $1 billion, and its success is largely following Tony's Zappos culture, the new culture for corporations today, making a positive change for us all. Great news.

In Las Vegas, the new Zappos headquarters moved into the old city hall, and Tony renovated it into floors of Zappos's new freeform business culture. I went on the tour of the new Zappos and was amazed at how everyone is equal in stature there—no big offices or fancy desks. Tony and the other executives have the same small cubicles everyone else does. They can decorate their own tiny spaces. I was told that Tony himself lives in a "tiny house." Or he did.

On each floor, there were large tables with chairs where employees were encouraged to mingle all day, talk over ways to improve the company, get and give ideas, and create, create, create. They had free snack bars on each floor that offered healthy treats for employees to eat whenever they felt the desire. There was a cafeteria with low prices and healthy foods, and they had their very own restaurant out front with low prices, drinks, and good food. Look for the companies today that are employing the Zappos culture, and you will find the kind of organization that values its employees, the truth, and what is best for all. I support these companies and drop the rest. This will make a huge change in the landslide toward the new paradigm. Thanks, Tony.

27. Bruce West, DC

This "tell it like it is" doctor, the founder of *Health Alert* (www. healthalert.com or 800-231-8063), is an expert in the use of Standard Process's top-quality supplements, made from real food. Originally, Royal Lee started Standard Process and wanted the supplements only sold through doctor's offices. That was idealistic, because most MDs know very little about nutrition and natural healing, and I recall how hard it used to be to find Standard Process products. Then I found Dr. West and *Health Alert*, and for a small membership fee, you receive *Doctor's A–Z Phytoceutical Guide*, a veritable encyclopedia of Dr. West's protocols using Standard Process products. He is very critical of medical mistakes out there and states that "medical errors are the number-one cause of death in America." I respect his knowledge, and I have used his protocols and Standard Process supplements with great success. I therefore consider *Health Alert* to be a truth tool you can use, and the Newsletter Dr. West authors.

28. Phyllis A. Balch, CNC

In every health-food store, the book *Prescription for Nutritional Healing: A Practical A-to-Z Reference to Drug-Free Remedies Using Vitamins, Minerals, Herbs & Food Supplements* has a stand to hold it so that you can use its over eight hundred pages of research your specific needs. I've had one at home for many years, and at the first sign I get that something is wrong, I go to this book first to see what it might be. Every home should have one. The information on each subject is based on a lot of years of experience, and the "Recommendations and Considerations" as well as the discussions are succinct but cover extensive knowledge. It really is America's number-one guide to natural healing information at a glance. You can find it in every health-food store, bookstore, and through Amazon. It is the best of all the choices.

CHAPTER 3

Spiritual Truth Heroes

These divine people—Buddha Maitreya, Oprah Winfrey, and Dr. Rev. Michael Bernard Beckwith each deserve a separate chapter devoted to how they kept me on my spiritual path while the hardships of pain and suffering challenged my body, kept my spirit alive and well, and gave me courage, faith, and hope.

Dr. Rev. Michael Bernard Beckwith

I listen to the CDs of Rev. Michael every day in my car, and they give me such a lift, as does the music in them that his wife, Rickie Byars Beckwith, orchestrates. It transcends what we think of as "church music" and becomes modern musical genius. I subscribe to the Wednesday and Sunday services CD copies and so receive new ones weekly—and do they ever motivate me, inspire me, and make me feel at one with the universe all at once.

I first saw Rev. Michael years ago in Sedona when he followed Dr. David Hawkins's introduction speech in a "Gift of the Shift" seminar. I already loved Dr. Hawkins and saw him at his lectures in Sedona, but when Rev. Michael came up to the microphone and started speaking, I sat up straighter. I'll never forget his saying right off, "Why try and change the old, broken systems when we can just walk into the new paradigm?" That has stayed with me ever since, and I try to practice it. When I get all flustered with the bureaucratic mess, I think on the higher plane of the new paradigm I live and think in, and all the rest disappears.

Rev. Michael founded the Agape International Spiritual Center in Culver City, California. His services are live-streamed all over the world. He talks about how we came here by choice to give our gifts to the world, not to see what we could "get." He also talks about how the Agape practitioners are "holding the field" because he is totally familiar with its quantum physics truths and importance in our lives today. So, forget the preachy past. Rev. Michael spent a lot of years at "A Course in Miracles" gatherings, and he has so little ego, has a divine sense of humor, and shines from the inside out.

I first visited the Agape center when I moved to Laguna Beach, not far from Culver City. Expecting to find a small church, the Agape Center is a cavernous commercial space that holds over a thousand people for each service. All of it's visitors come to hear Rev. Michael's incredible wisdom and listen to Rickie's music that rocks the whole place with her talent, the house choir, and famous musical guests. The energy of love is palpable in these services, in this modern Spiritual expression that only Agape delivers today, with an unbeatable holistic verve. Pure energy.

I had just listened to *The Mysteries of Water* CD and felt it was so important that I wanted to give it to Rev. Michael somehow. But when I saw this huge service, the only thing I could think to do was put it in the collection plate as it passed along with my offering. Oh, well, I thought. Two weeks later, I got a call from Sherry at Agape, who said, "Thank you, thank you!" She told me about how they'd all watched it and loved it, adding that if I had any other things for them I should contact her personally. Well, that felt great! I had "connected," despite thinking I'd never hear what happened with that CD, and that's the way I feel when I listen to Michael—connected, because he is connected, deeply and profoundly.

He doesn't tell you how to live like most religious leaders but rather how to think, how to find the truth in things eternal, not worldly, and how to quit the addiction to mediocrity in favor of practicing excellence. His CDs add such wisdom and joy to my life and support to my soul in his spiritual truths. He is a real hero in this world today for lifting us out of the garbage can of "reality" shows and into a high plane of consciousness and awareness. Our connection with others on that plane is strength and oneness, not the conflict and division of false ego-based beliefs that harm.

How Rickie brings the Agape choir and house band plus the musical talents in Los Angeles to play great music for the services is also very cool. It makes you want to get up and dance! I think of that Methodist preacher I grew up listening to but not hearing, and the choir music I couldn't hear either, and see the difference between the light of Agape and the dark ages of organized religion. I sidestep all that now in favor of the new paradigm of love and service in conscious awareness, mastering my ego so that it doesn't master me, witnessing compassion, beauty, and joy daily with Rev. Beckwith's CDs and Rickie's original songs.

Recently I listened to a CD where Don Miguel Ruiz spoke at Agape, talking about his new book. (He wrote *The Four Agreements*, a favorite of mine.) He talked about how his having a big heart attack changed his life. He said that the same conflict exists in all of us but that it isn't between "good and bad" but between "truth and lies," mentioning how superstitions (lies) are the underlying reason for wars and violence because people feel they must defend them. I thought about this for a long time and about how truth was always my goal. Now I was even more committed to it, and I had to learn to love without conditions.

With each of the two CDs I receive each week comes an index-sized card with Rev. Michael's "Meditative Thought" on one side ("Enthusiasm is our passport to our inner search," one of them begins) and Affirmations on the other ("A grand vision of possibility is the blueprint for my life!"). I love reading them out loud. I pass these and the CDs on to others, along with Michael's books and other Agape information at www.agapelive.com. One can also call Alice's Quiet Mind Bookstore (310-348-1266) or the office (310-348-1250). Contributions to spreading the Agape word globally make me feel good. Edwene Gaines said to support the people who support you spiritually so that you will have something to give others and stay whole.

Oprah Winfrey

Holy smoke, what can I say about this truth heroine magnifique? Is she not the most beautiful, evolved person on this planet? Oprah's "Super Soul Sunday" is a gift to us all as she interviews top-of-the-world spiritual stargate authors and speakers as only she can, finding the deep spiritual truths of their souls, sans ego, false pride, and arrogance. She is the most real, likeable, best spoken, and best overall interviewer. Her core is pure, and despite enormous pressures, her rules are simple. Her talks with spiritual people make me feel warm and safe all over, as if I were ten years old in my jammies listening to God. Knowing there are people like her and her guests in this world to multiply my faith and help me heal is the highest gift. Even a Nobel wouldn't suffice to thank this brilliant, balanced, funny, dedicated, authentic spiritual powerhouse of giving, giving, and more giving.

I've been watching all of Oprah's TV shows over many years to learn more about behavior, humanity, self-respect, respect for others, and loving myself and everyone else. I learned forgiveness and to sit on my ego like she does, even when challenged by unruly guests. During all my travails, Oprah was there to tune me into her faith and hope, and I thank this lady of goodness and greatness with all my heart. Oprah's one hundred percent honesty and truth seeking is what kept her free of therapy despite her rough start, and I emulated that. She is the ultimate role model for females in this world and the others as well.

It shouldn't surprise us that Oprah's book *What I Know for Sure* calibrates at 960 on the Map of Consciousness when the highest truth/consciousness score is 1,000. I would say that Oprah is one of the most evolved people on the planet and has stayed true to the truth, seeing her wealth and power follow due to her perfect alignment with God/source, truth, compassion, and wisdom. I love watching her on each and every show, because if she can do it, so can I. Only God can thank Oprah enough.

His Holiness Buddha Maitreya

Of course, your first question is "Who?" This is a "who" who scores 1,000, the highest score on the Map of Consciousness, who is the only living incarnation of the Maitreya (teacher) Buddha, and who founded the magnificent Church of Shambhala Monastery fairly recently in Kelseyville, California, north of San Francisco.

I visited many lectures at the Creative Life Center's events in Sedona, and at one of them I purchased a CD that my pendulum picked out called *Archangels of Heaven*. I put it in my car's CD player, and when I heard it, I was mystified—it sounded like nothing I'd ever heard before. On the long drive home to Prescott, I let it play over and over. It made me feel so ethereal, so peaceful and accepting, calm and joyous, free to be me. It was the only CD in my car for that whole year because I never tired of it, and it always made me feel so content. The voice chants, the music with bells and chimes, washed over me like a cleansing of soul and spirit. When I had so much on my plate in the business of owning commercial real estate, this CD took me to a higher plane where that stress was way distant and unimportant as the haunting sounds flooded my body with spiritual blessings.

Toward the end of the CD, the voice's haunting lines were so magnificent that I could never write them all down. Here are some fragments, all in a powerful voice of firm love:

Let the forces of life bring illumination to mankind...may the humanity of good will go everywhere...let power attend the efforts of the great ones...let the lords of liberation issue forth...let the souls of mankind awaken to the light...come forth, oh mighty one, to restore the plan on earth...from the center where the will of God is known, the will to save is here, the love to spread the word is here. Come forth, oh mighty one, the rule of evil now must end; seal the door where evil dwells...the sons of man are one, and I am one with them...

It just made me want to fall into his strength and become one in his army of goodness and light.

Remarkably, I never even looked to see who produced this CD; I just accepted it as mine. That is, until I decided to take it out to see, and unfortunately I ruined it because my fingers were sticky from lunch. Then I had to find out how to get a new copy, was how I found His Holiness Buddha Maitreya. It was his CD, his voice, his music and bells.

When I called to find a replacement for the CD I'd ruined, they told me I could get one at the Soul Center Store in Sedona in the Hillside Shopping Center. When I got there, I saw a giant, four-foot-long clear crystal hanging near the window along with all these magnificent pieces of what seemed like jumbo jewelry from a land of giants. With a feeling of overpowering beauty, I saw Buddha Maitreya's healing tools made of precious metals and colored crystals in shapes so geometric and familiar and yet so strange to me. I asked the Ani (nun) who greeted me how to choose from all the colors. She said the ones you like best are the right ones. The Anis helped me choose tools that are available now at www.BuddhaMaitreyaHealingtools. com (the Sedona store is closed), including the seven CDs they told me to play all the time, including *Archangels of Heaven*, and I did. I used their Metatron mat system to lie on for all the time I could—I even slept on it. I played all seven of Buddha Maitreya's CDs relentlessly; I used their Etheric Weaver for my pendulum and held a Vajra in each hand while lying on the mat. I hung the Solar Cross over my bed and wore a blessed beautiful crystal, gold, and copper pendant for protection. I was so sick for so long, I would try anything.

In just fourteen days, I jumped out of bed, looked at my little dog, and said, "Rudy, we're going to the beach!" I went directly to my home office and called Loew's Beach Hotel in Santa Monica to make a reservation for a week starting the following day. Tell me about miracles! I hadn't been to a beach for many years! But since then, I have never looked back to the helpless ten years of on-and-off chronic fatigue—and did we ever have a great time at the beach laughing and playing. I plopped Rudy into the water for the first time, and everything felt so fine. I didn't spend a second thinking about it, as if everything before the beach was already ancient history.

I could write volumes about this soul-truth holy man, but look online at his healing tools, see them visually, and read the descriptions of how they work, and you'll feel a glow come over you. Don't faint over the prices, these are gold or silver plated, the finest crystal, made custom for you by hand by the monks at the monastery. This is an investment for a lifetime. I couldn't put a price on how these very tools that use sacred geometry got me alive again in just fourteen days. Everyone asks me about my Buddha Maitreya pendant, and they are so attracted to it energetically. Call 877-444-SOUL (7685) for a catalog. There is so much to say about the stunning architecture of the Shambhala Monastery—domes and pyramids based on geomancy, depicting the creation, the maintaining, and the evolution of the planet; the cosmos, the system of life, and God—everything. They say that when we build with sacred design and work with vibration and healing and faith, we're actually working to heal the soul. When we apply geomancy, such as building a temple, we are actually building a place where the energy of the soul can be collected, stored, and placed into the earth. The earth radiates more love, more kindness, more humanity, less war."

The seven buildings of the Shambhala Monastery have three levels, with the first floor underground. From 1994, His Holiness has been supporting monasteries, sacred sites, and health clinics around the world, and he is here only to serve and love. Today, the monastery offers sophisticated treatments for the public, retreats, and more at this idyllic site overlooking a lake. Not enough can be said about the spiritual plane His Holiness and his wife, the monastery, and the tools offer us in healing truths with the highest vibrational advances, especially all the love inside that he gives away nearly every waking hour. I listened to the CD entitled *Metatronics: Quantum Physics of the Science of God*, for instance. On it, someone asked him if he designed all these tools. He said, "No, I just knew." His Holiness was born in Oregon in 1951, and I'm excited to follow what he will do in the future. His blessing dissolves past karma too.

This concludes my special chapter for spiritual truth heroes, featuring three mighty personas that kept me on the spiritual path once I'd found it through all their love gifts for us with no agendas—just pure consciousness, pure love, and pure service. Thank you, God.

CHAPTER 4

True Health Helpers

———————

These were all big discovery winners for me:

1. UVLRx–Intravenous Light Treatment

This latest greatest treatment machine is beyond belief. Discovered at an integrative cancer conference, my doctors at Partners for Health Care Naturally here in Prescott, AZ have already purchased a second one (at $40,000 each) because of demand, especially in treating chronic conditions with pain and inflammation, including cancer, Lyme, autoimmunity disorders, infections, and fatigue.

The first time I received a one-hour treatment, I felt twenty years younger that very same day. It was a miracle, I swear, and I think of it as the "ultimate" treatment. I hope you have the UVLRx available in your area too, because the demand has already gone to Europe. Check www.uvlrx.com to find UVLRx you can get to (or call 844-885-7979). It works as your blood is exposed to various wavelengths of light where the catheter and needle go into your arm. In the hour it takes for all your blood to pass by this light, there are three wavelengths of light:

UVA—Eradicates pathogens (no Herxheimer or extreme reaction)

RED—Upregulates cell bioenergetics, lowers inflammation, bolsters immunity for more antibodies and to repair cells
GREEN—Improves blood flow and circulation

I did five of these treatments in a row to sort of clean up the terrain with many pathogens, and I have "tune-ups" as needed periodically. I waited six months before I had another one. I do one or two as needed now.

UV light is a powerful antimicrobial agent against pathogens and inflammation in this LED light intervention. It's safe, simple, and effective. See the education video on their site.

2. Angioprim–Treatment for Arterial Blockages

I found Angioprim years ago, after a friend with heart problems met the inventor, also a resident of Las Vegas, and raved about it to me. Now I'm raving to you.

My father died at forty-six of a heart attack. Only twelve at the time, I remember that it was four in the morning as I watched the Dad I loved so much writhing in pain in his bed, as Mom was calling the ambulance. I never saw him again, and that was the biggest heartbreak of my life. So, I had early clues that I should pay attention to my heart, and I was right that I had problems. I later found atherosclerosis repeatedly coming up on my biofeedback machine, along with cardiomyopathy and other heart issues. This wonderful remedy has worked great for cleaning out my arteries over the past ten years, chelating out the plaque from my high cholesterol, or calcium, whatever plaque sticks. I originally did the full twenty-eight-day treatment for a major cleanout, which means taking the little Angioprim half bottle and a tall glass of the right juice and sipping it slowly before eating or drinking anything else every morning. I really enjoyed doing that; it slowed me down and gave me permission to lollygag around in my robe and read while I sipped. You wait a half hour to eat and that's it, the Roto-Rooter goes to work.

I have done tune-ups with Angioprim ever since, taking it again as needed, sometimes for three days or, if I wait too long, longer. Symptoms of arterial blockages are listed on their site (www.angioprim.com). The ingredients in Angioprim are Caysine (synthetic amino), Lysine (amino), and Cysteine (amino). After the treatments, you do need to restore minerals in your body with supplements, and you're good to go until you need to clean out again. From having Lyme disease, I learned that health does not mean being devoid of pathogens. Nobody is. Rather, it's "managing" to be optimum, using all these tools, and continuing to learn.

3. Amethyst Biomat 7000mx by Richway International, Inc.

When I first bought my Biomat thirteen years ago, they were made of jade crystals, and mine is still working fine. They have since been switched to amethyst, which I have to assume is even better. Through my entire life, I've had muscle spasms so severe that the tension was impossible to bear (Pyroluria). Alcohol was the best treatment, but alas, I had to go to work. I tried muscle relaxers (Formula 303 worked best), but when I met a healer who distributed the Biomat, I was intrigued. She warmed up the sample Biomat, and I tried it. I was thrilled. Its far-infrared rays heat the gemstone crystals and produce healthy negative ions from natural tourmaline (another gemstone). An EMF interceptor reduces any electromagnetic waves, too.

I never wanted to get off the Biomat, and so I bought one. Now, when my friends try mine, they never want to get off it either! The relaxation is so (lovingly) warm and goes so deep, I even use it to warm me up when I'm cold to the bone. Heat kills pathogens too, although they don't mention this, and I also use the highest heat from the very sophisticated controller to sweat out toxins. It makes your blood circulate and produces negative ions the way waterfalls and oceans, mountains and forests do. Biomats come in various sizes and prices, each accompanied by a certificate of gem identification authenticating the amethyst, which is expensive but will last forever, so what a great investment. My whole life I wasn't able to relax because of all the muscle tension due to sports, stress, Lyme, and Pyroluria. The whole family will want to use it, trust me. You'll be drawing straws. Count your dog in, too.

4. Ozonator–Ozone Generator

Dr. Clark's books introduced me to ozonators, and I purchased one to help me clean foods, ozonate water, infuse into olive oil, and use as an antibacterial. They are in the air cleaners I use and work on molds, odors, and sterilization—a must if you have pets. The ozonator with the long tube can sterilize all your fruits and vegetables in a sink full of water, and after air drying, they'll last longer and stay fresher.

The most important story I have about using an ozonator (the tube kind) is a dental experience in Mexico. After my mercury tested the highest ever, I had all my mercury fillings and caps replaced in Las Vegas by the top dentist recommended by the Nevada clinic, which I've already mentioned. It surprised me that I didn't feel better after all that, but I said, "Oh, well" and felt I'd done all I could do. Eleven years later, all that dental work started chipping and cracking, as composite replacements were new then. I got an estimate for replacing all this work, and they wanted a staggering $25,000. I heard about Mexican dentists doing a great job and called one that was recommended in Tijuana, with good credentials. He had me send my X-rays and then told me he would do it for $10,000, and I agreed. He warned me that he and his colleagues in San Diego were finding black mold under the composite fillings of people who had their mercury amalgams removed. Mold is my most serious allergy, and I have no resistance to fungal infection, which I later learned was because my mother had it too, so prenatally it became part of me.

I flew from Las Vegas to San Diego, where I went for four weeks, renting a car and crossing the border to find the dentist's office in Tijuana, doing one quadrant of my mouth each week. After it was over, he told me he'd found that eighty percent of my fillings had black mold underneath. To avoid my having this mold again, he recommended using an ozonator, mine is the size of a fishing tackle box, to sterilize everything inside my mouth. He used his ozonator on everything he drilled out as well as everything he was adding back in—caps, composite, glue, and so on. It all got carefully ozonated. He never had me rinse my mouth with water, either, very important.

When I finished the dental makeover, I had a huge Herxheimer reaction and was sick as a dog for two months suffering with flu-like symptoms. But after that, I started to really get better now. The mold issue is still not known here in the United States, so I bring my own ozonator in to the dentist if I need a minor repair, like my chipped front tooth. That was fifteen years ago. I haven't had a cavity since, my lava crowns are still cool, and I'd recommend a Mexican dentist too, if you're in proximity—and an ozonator.

5. Soloflex–Whole-Body Vibration Platform

When I was in bed with chronic fatigue for so long, I had no energy to exercise. After being into yoga and tennis for years before I got sick, I was feeling my muscles turn to flab. Then www.soloflex.com came up somehow, a vibrational platform you stand on while you work out with weights that can be used for seniors' resistance strength training or to increase a workout's effect by standing on it. I remembered using chi machines, so I lay on the floor and put my feet up on it or sat on it, because that was all I could do then, and it helped my poor circulation from being in bed all the time, picked me up, and helped me feel that I was doing something for exercise. Today, I use it for strength training when I'm not outside walking or doing another exercise, For those who aren't able to do more at this stage of their recovery, it can help a lot to reduce pain, anxiety, and depression, like it did for me.

6. Orgone Energy Pyramids–Orgone Energy

Orgone is the universal life force, the basic building block of all organic and inorganic matter on the planet, also called chi, mana, prana, life energy, or the force. The accumulator was layers of organic material and metals; in resin, they can be made into cones, pyramids, pendants, charger plates, etc. It changes the state of energy to balanced, healthy energy from negative energy. When orgonite is near any source of EMF (electromagnetic field or electro-smog) radiation, it will attract it and absorb it. Since EMFs interfere with biological systems, it works for protection of cell phones and even helps dissolve stored or blocked past experiences in the body. Orgonite makes positive vibes from negative electrical devices within three feet (www.orgoniteinfo.com) using scalar wave technology. Microwave radiation sautés your DNA; orgonite repairs it.

They add gorgeous quartz and metals to small pyramids and cones, making them look almost like jewelry. (Etsy.com has a nice collection.) I use orgonite cones around all my heavy-duty EMFs like the computer, printer, TVs, and so on. They can help with Geopathic Stressors and the effects of cell towers, and I bought a tabletop energizer from www.quwave.com to energize food and water with scalar waves and Orgone chi energy. I have noticed even more energy since I've been using the four-inch-square device on my spring water. Sometimes I put the words *love* and *thank you* on a paper underneath, thanks to Dr. Emoto.

7. Trifield Meter 100XE–EMF Measurement

Years ago, as I was getting sicker and sicker, I read about EMFs, or electromagnetic fields, and how they affect your health negatively. Recommendations were coming out that you should call your local power company and have them check your house for electric read-outs, so I did. I was in Las Vegas, and there was a power-company easement in the backyard behind my house and my art studio. These nice fellows from the power company told me that under 2 hertz was safe for humans, so we started their tests with the outside easement area of buried power lines. The reading was 10 hertz right over the easement, really dangerous to human health. Then we went into my studio about ten feet away, and it measured 2.5 hertz there. We got to the center of the house which was 0.06 hertz, which they said was normal and as it should be.

Inside they started showing me how high different appliances are—computers, gadgets, and so on—and they said to keep my distance from them, as their readouts on the Trifield were astronomical. When they left, I tossed a lot of the gadgets. I was so impressed with this testing that I bought the Trifield Meter so I could measure electric, magnetic, and radio waves myself. Later, when I ordered DirecTV via satellite, I wondered if that changed anything. When I got my Trifield Meter on the case, the 0.06 "normal" went to 1.06, a whole hertz unit higher. That made me realize I had to stop bringing in more EMFs. I needed things to stay under 2.

That was long ago and far away from all that's available today—Wi-Fi, routers, Bluetooth, wireless—that passes through walls and isn't turned off at night. And you are exposed to your neighbors' EMFs too. It's like layering radiation fields.

The Trifield 100XE (www.trifield.com) is about $145 today and well worth it. When I moved into a new house later on, I found a great big closet that I made my vitamin and health pantry. After putting everything into this closet, I thought to get out the Trifield, and sure enough, it went bonkers. I kept retesting the closet and then the wall of the house behind it, which also registered very high. I finally realized that this center wall held all the electricals to the whole house and everything else, so out came all the vitamins I would have "fried" had I left them there. That space became a linen closet again. But you can see the size of mistakes we can make.

Microwave ovens are 2.45 billion hertz inside, and as they age, the seal loosens and leaks can occur. Besides, they change the molecular structure of food, which leads to illness later.

Trifield measures all three electromagnetic pollutions: magnetic, electric, and radio microwaves. They're another fun device for health truth for us Medical Detectives. They give you news you can use to find out if power lines, cell towers, cell phones, smart phones, smart meters, or underground pipes are in your home energy unit along with all the appliances, computers, printers, and so on inside. Remember, they shouldn't add up to over 2 hertz total.

If they do, you can remedy the situation with other helpers. For example, www.safespaceprotection.com has GeoResonators to clear and protect the earth energy, clear Geopathic Stress zones, and transmute the negative impacts of ground current. They also have EMF adapters for Wi-Fi, routers, wireless, computers, and so on. As you know, we are being bombarded with new bits of technology every day, so it's good to test your home with the Trifield Meter and defend your health as necessary. You'll feel the difference.

CHAPTER 5

Important Truth Considerations

These subjects are unknown to most people, including professionals, and I'm adding in the ones that I found played a big role in my illness recovery. Please follow them online for more information if you need better understandings of their importance.

1. Geopathic Stress and Ley Lines

Geopathic Stress is caused by the natural Ley Lines that cover the planet in a huge grid. Different ones affect us in different ways. The Hartmann Cross, for example, is a cancer causer. The Szent-Georgi Cross causes blood sugar problems. Curry Lines affect the body's electrical systems; the Water Cross keeps your immunity at bay and causes illness over time, which is what happened to me. I built a home in Las Vegas over a former water-drainage path. One day, I found a chip in the second-floor banister, in the paint from the inside wood, and found termites. The exterminator told me that where there are termites, there is water, and he traced the water to under the house. The Water Cross Geopathic Stress factor that had made me so sick in the twelve years I lived there was suddenly revealed. I had to move—and the sooner, the better.

I went to a seminar where two German MDs were discussing cancer treatment. Ulrike Banis, MD, and her husband, another MD, said they had found that one hundred percent of their cancer patients slept in Geopathic Stress zones, and if the patients refused to move their beds, they wouldn't treat them. Their book and others discuss this.

I use the pendulum now, or rods, to test for these Geopathic Stress zones. Where they cross over each other is especially significant. They are usually only about three feet wide, and you can find the direction they are coming from and going to. Where you see what I call "cancer trees," those that have tumors or lumps all over them, they are in a Geopathic Stress zone, and if you look around and line up with other trees like it, a lot of weeds, and other clues, you will see signs of the path they are on. Learning to be aware of things in your environment is really interesting. These zones go straight up to the sky; you can't go high enough to get out of them, and high-rises will have them in the same place on the top floor as on the first floor. First place to test is your bed.

In Germany, you can't build a new building without the government checking the site for Geopathic Stress, and you may not be able to get permits to build. In the United States, nobody ever heard of it. Well, this is another truth tool. Read up about Ley Lines and this grid and what these things that come from the earth can do to make us sick. This truth tool should be taught in schools so that kids become aware of the factors that could influence their health and behavior. The most significant places are those in which we spend the most time, especially the bed, favorite chair, or desk you work at all day or sit in school. A Geopathic Stress factor can be crossing through them. Usually they cross where the illness is in the body. You can use rods to dowse for these if you're doing big areas. Energy testing is a life saver.

My biofeedback tests kept indicating "Hartmann Cross," and I was testing with my pendulum (P) around this black leather recliner

I sit in to read and got yes, but I couldn't find a path of it. Then it dawned on me that the hydraulic-lift apparatus to recline it had to be causing the cancer-causing Hartmann Cross. So, I tried mounting my Orgone pyramid armies, but they weren't strong enough to fix it. This was the same as my brother's office chair and its hydraulic lift, but one Orgone cone two feet from it fixed that effect on it, I saw after I tested on my Trifield. So, this chair of mine is a current challenge, because if I can't find a fix, it will have to find its way out of here. Test any hydraulic chairs. I have another leather loveseat that reclines at the touch of electric buttons, and I don't get any Geopathic Stress read-outs from it. It plugs into a wall socket.

I also prefer leather furniture over upholstered furniture, which gives off formaldehyde, and I use air cleaners. A friend had me come over with my Trifield Meter to test her home after her husband was diagnosed with cancer, and I told her about the bed story. Sure enough, the outside wall right behind the MBR bed on her husband's side had all the electrical equipment for their huge swimming pool mounted on it. Then I saw his cell-phone charger next to his side of the bed on the nightstand (they should be as far away as you can put them)—right next to a clock radio! I would call that a perfect recipe for cancer, but then I also found Ley Lines crossing over on the bed for good measure. She moved the bed, but you can see how invisible the problem can be just due to lack of information about truth tool testing and Geopathic Stress.

2. Miasms

Miasms were perceived by the famous Dr. Hahnemann, the discoverer of homeopathy, as the parasitical nature of infections or contagious diseases, including syphilis, gonorrhea, leprosy, tuberculosis, cholera, typhus, typhoid, and chronic diseases in general. There are miasms for cancer, polio, and psora, and I have seen newer ones for AIDS, ringworm, and miasmatic allergies today as bacteria and microorganisms become the agents connected with the manifestation of diseases reflecting the miasms.

The word *miasma* means stain, pollution, or defilement. The germ of disease, or microorganisms, bacteria, fungi, viruses, protozoa, parasites, can be the cause of disease. We call these pathogens. Miasmatic predisposition and susceptibility involve DNA and influence subsequent generations. According to Dr. Hahnemann, the number of miasms will gradually increase and will affect the predisposition of a child from the parents. Some disease conditions develop when miasmatic states are combined and produce the most complicated chronic illnesses. Dr. Hahnemann considered psora the most ancient, although syphilis and gonorrhea have also been around for thousands of years.

Dr. Hahnemann thought suppression of these, say using antibiotics, plus vaccinations, created the complex mixtures of diseases today, and I think I've proven him right. My biofeedback machine shows I have almost all of the miasms, which explains why I have had so many coinfections with Lyme. As I zap the frequency of one, up comes another the next time I use it. Lyme is a spirochete or corkscrew-like form, and so is syphilis, and I have discovered from all those I've put on my machine that Lyme disease only gets fully manifested in those who have the syphilis miasm.

Others may show it but may not be very sick or in wheelchairs. Lyme can show up in everyone since the government let it escape years ago and today may be dropping it in chemtrails. I see the many coinfections of Lyme go up and down in acuteness as well along with the miasms, so it appears this miasm is connected with the disease, like Lyme and syphilis. From watching what these pathogens do on me when I test every week or so, I am certain these various pathogens cooperate, communicate, and share in the host's resources.

Our genealogy interests today may discover ancestors who died of bubonic plague, for example, and passed down the miasmatic predisposition. Today, most of us have mixed miasms. In Misha Norland's book *Signatures, Miasms, AIDS*, she writes, "Because inoculation inhibits or distorts the primary manifestation of childhood diseases, it interferes with the natural tendency of the body to throw out miasmatic tendencies. In other words, the practice is suppressive, the payoff is chronic disease in place of acute disease."

I see on my machine how often my childhood vaccinations still come up in "acute" high numbers as interfering with my health, along with the tetanus shot I had to have in order to travel to India years ago. (What children receive today is unexplainable.) Clients on my machine all show trouble from childhood vaccinations.

Different books on miasms list them in different ways. When I saw one adding ringworm, a particularly nasty memory surfaced for me because I'd had ringworm when I was nine, and they had to shave my head. I have no conscious memory of what that did to me in school. I would think there would have been jokes, but maybe sympathy as well. I don't have any resistance to fungal infections. As I mentioned, my mother had had it, so it was in my blueprint? They couldn't fix it in New Jersey, so Mom took me to New York University (NYU), where they were doing a study, and they got rid of it. Of course, it took a year for my hair to return, and after that, the NYU study followed me all over the globe with questionnaires every year, even when I moved to Greece. They had a placebo group and a group that got radiation, and since they followed me everywhere until I was thirty-five, and because I got letters from them to watch for thyroid cancer, I finally called NYU to see which group I was in. Luckily, I was in the placebo group. I was glad when they finally stopped it, since it made me feel like there was something they were not telling me. Why else would they have been following this study for so long? So, I of course thought they were right to add ringworm miasm to the list. Other books on miasms include

Indications of Miasm by Dr. Harimohon Choudhury and *Miasms: Their Effects on Human Organism* by Raju and Raaji Subramanian. Sadly, western allopathic medicine has ignored this very important aspect of disease.

Lyme and mold go together, as the illustrious expert Dr. Dietrich Klinghardt, MD, taught me via his articles on www.klinghardtneurobiology.com under "Articles." When you treat one, you have to treat them both, or you won't win, he maintains. I also have the huge mold allergy and therefore toss out any food that's been in the refrigerator more than four days. Even if you don't see the mold, it's there. I also have Candida, my next subject. Do you?

3. Candida

Over twenty species of Candida yeasts exist—Candida is the most overlooked cause of many problems—and still MDs refuse to address it, probably because they never studied it and don't know about it. This is in the fungi-mold-yeast group and has many forms, be it *albicans, tropicalis, pseudotropicales, rugosa, utilis, parapsilosis, krusei, lusitaniae*, and so on. An Italian MD wrote a book on how *Candida albicans* causes cancer. I remember years ago when I would suddenly crave alcohol and binge drink. My friend owned a raw food restaurant, and I told her I was at a loss about what drove me to do that, saying I was already in the car on my way to the store to get a bottle of wine before I knew what I was doing. Then I'd drink down what felt like enough wine and just suddenly stop without even finishing the bottle. The next day, I'd hate myself for the fuzzy hangover and pour out what was left. There seemed to be a set point, and when I reached it, I quit.

She asked me if I had Candida.

"What's Candida?" I asked.

"It's the beast that makes you drink—and a lot of other things."

I later found Joan Matthews Larson's book 7 *Weeks to Emotional Healing*, as I mentioned in the chapter on truth heroes, and located the Candida questionnaire. I tested for it along with Pyroluria, my next subject, and both scores were extremely high. One of the questions in the list was, "Do you crave alcoholic beverages?" I wish I could reproduce this terrific questionnaire for you, but copyright and Random House say no. Others were, "Have you had ringworm?" "Have you taken antibiotics?" "Do you use birth-control pills?" The list went on. All my answers were yes, plus what I learned later about having no resistance to any fungal infections.

The Candida Diet is out there now, and adding wild oregano oil, caprylic acid, kyolic garlic, citrus-seed extract, and acidophilus on top of that along with 2000mg. of methylsulfonylmethane (MSM) a day, plus Gymnema sylvestre and Undecylenic Acid, berberine, and HCl should work to keep it in check. Test each with P to find what is best for you, then if in combination, and how many of each (capsules or mgs. or powder). I find I am usually deficient in sulfur and the MSM provides that, which has many benefits in addition to detoxing and Candida. Since we each have a little Candida in us naturally, we can't eradicate it completely but a good keep it in check diet helps. I don't eat bleu cheese, mushrooms, peanuts, or vinegar, but I do cheat on peanuts, melons, and cheeses occasionally., because they have other things I need. Candida could put me on an emotional roller coaster when I was younger and didn't have the recipe to control it, and my hormones were a lot more active. I don't know of one book that lists all the kinds of Candida that show up for me. People's research extends as far as the book *The Yeast Connection*, and then they quit. Big mistake for this heavy hitter in illness and disease. Luckily, the new magazine *"What Doctors Don't Tell You"* whose editors are Lynne McTaggart, the famed author of one of the earliest books I read on Quantum Physics, *The Field*, now famous and classic, and Bryan Hubbard, are bringing this to the forefront. The December 2016 issue has the cover story *Lose the Bloat- A real solution to Candida*. I was immensely pleased to find Lynn McTaggart on the scene and this new magazine that is long overdue to put the truth out there. Always test articles with your truth tools to know if they are accurate and true. We are in our toddler state of knowledge about health, so we need to check the source and calibrate it on the Map of Consciousness scale before we start doing any protocols we read about in magazines with so many authors. Lynn says her Candida was how this magazine was formed, and God Bless her for doing something about it! Me too!

4. Food Allergies–Lectins and Salycilates

Food allergies are a huge factor in health, and I learned that what I thought were food sensitivities or allergies kept changing on my biofeedback tests. I blamed it on wearing out my liver with supplements, until I found *The Lectin Report* online and did some more research. I found out that lectins were my problem and were causing me many awful effects that I'd thought were from other pathogens. I learned that I may be lectin toxic due to genetics, intensity of exposure, failure of immune factors to protect me from them, viral infection, bacterial infection, or leaky gut. Lectin sensitivity can manifest as arthritis, allergies, asthma, high cholesterol, atherosclerosis, congestive heart failure, high blood pressure, diabetes, low blood sugar, hyperinsulinemia, chronic fatigue, fibromyalgia, all forms of IBS, Crohn's, Colitis, Celiac, chronic Candida, repeated gut infections, malabsorption, autoimmune diseases, thyroiditis, Lupus, MS, Parkinson's, dementia, Alzheimer's, Autism, ADD/ADHD, schizophrenia, cancer (several kinds, including breast), hypercortisolemia, hypothyroid, adrenal insufficiency, post-viral syndrome, posttraumatic stress syndrome, post-polio syndrome, obesity, hormonal imbalances like low testosterone, low DHEA, PMS, and perimenopause symptoms.

I hope that got your attention—do your research on this to find out if it is a major player in your illness too. Because lectins are found in many foods, I take a lectin blocker to block it when I eat. Highest lectins are found in gluten/wheat and all grains. Wheat has been genetically modified drastically, increasing lectin to a level ninety percent higher than our grandparents' wheat. Most people would be better off without gluten today, and it is a big additive now. Stress can also contribute to the attaching of lectins, and food additives, fillers, and thickeners can intensify their effect.

Beans, lentils, green peas, corn, walnuts, soy, bananas, peanuts, dairy, oils from soy or peanut, chicken, seafood, fruits, eggs, potatoes, tomatoes, eggplant, peppers, avocado, cabbage, Jerusalem artichoke, goji berry, and other foods can have high amounts. There are lists online showing higher and lower amounts, but I've found it very difficult to get the same answers with my pendulum on, say, a kind of fruit or vegetable. It depends on where it was grown, how it was processed, and so on. So, it was very hard for me to use the lists for more than the top groups, like grains and beans, nuts, seeds, and soy, and I find tomatoes are high. It's easier to take the lectin blockers and enjoy food again. There are three lectin blockers I know of. The illustrious Dr. D'Adamo's product called Deflect has slightly different formulas for each blood type, on his website www.4yourtype.com online. Then there are Dr. Cutler's Ultimate Lectin Defense by True Health (1-800-746-4513) and Lectin Lock by Vitamin Research Products (1-800-877-2447). Phenols are in all foods also, and some are sensitive to phenols and need to test for this also. There are Phenol blockers available. My only concern is whether the blocking is part of "malabsorption" that makes even fewer nutrients absorb. Malabsorption comes with the territory of several causes, like Celiac Disease, etc. and I have "starvation" coming up on my machine at times, so always ask P for the answers.

Salicylates are another phenol, aspirin being one and a good tester. If you're allergic to aspirin, you'll know. This information was paramount to my recovery because I lost so much energy over lectin sensitivity for a lot of years. I was a picky eater as a child, and P agrees that I was born with it. It had taken its toll on me with malabsorption until I found the blockers. Phenol sensitivity is a question to ask, as even supplements may have high phenol content, as I found with Milk Thistle for example. Despite many liver problems, it never got P saying "yes" it was good for me, and I didn't know why until I learned about my phenol sensitivity. Another example of why no one protocol is good for everyone! You must be able to test your body yourself to make your best choices based on the truth tools.

5. Pyroluria

I know you've never heard of this. Neither did I before that Larson book 7 *Weeks to Emotional Healing* mentioned earlier, and I tested for it and got high numbers. Because of the deficiencies it causes in vitamin B6 and zinc alone, this molecule made by the kidney, or pyrrole, was a "psychiatric disaster." I'll never forget that line from Larson's book.

If you have extreme muscle spasms, anxiety, muscle tension, or anxiety and can't relax, doubly so under stress, you may want to investigate Pyroluria, as it is called today, or mauve factor or heme-pyrrole. If you have poor dream recall, you are deficient in B6; this is one clear clue. Others are stitches in your side when you run and an aversion to eating breakfast. The questionnaire in Larson's *Seven Weeks to Sobriety* includes this, as anxiety and tension are relieved by alcohol or drugs. Hence my binge drinking was for relief of my combined Candida and Pyroluria making me crazy.

Dietrich Klinghardt, MD, gives the best description of Pyroluria in an hour-long YouTube presentation, and he connects pyrroles with Lyme disease, as most Lymees have it. But you don't have to have Lyme, so it can be either way. The treatment is supplementation to fix the deficiencies, which can take time to catch up but will make you feel an enormous difference. For instance, it took me two years for me to catch up with vitamin B6 deficiency, even with high daily doses. There are questionnaires for Pyroluria online, and in Larson's books.

Conditions associated with Pyroluria include allergies, ADD/ADHD, porphyria, Asperger's, Autism, bipolar disorder, depression, Down syndrome, epilepsy, lung cancer, neurosis, Tourette's, alcoholism, and substance abuse. You'll find more detailed information online as well, but leaky gut is widespread in Pyroluria people and drives pyrrole levels up; so does zinc deficiency, heavy metals, and stress. Pyrroles are classified as nerve poisons affecting your nerves and brain. It's believed to decrease heme levels in people, but the medical establishment ignores it because fixing it requires only natural supplements, not drugs. It can cause low blood volume and hypovolemic shock, which comes up for me on my biofeedback tests sometimes, and can be fatal.

Bone biopsies show deficiencies in B6 (PSP), zinc, manganese, lithium, calcium, magnesium, omega 6, glutathione, taurine, biotin, arachidonic acid, B vitamins, and low-count white blood cells that interfere with the methylation cycle. I take a supplement for methylation. There are usually mold problems along with pyrroles, plus an inability of the body to make vitamin B-1, thiamine, for the thymus for immunity, so you can see how important this factor can be for health. I would say this was the worst part of my illness, because the inner tension and nervous exhaustion were physically insurmountable on top of my stressful commercial real estate career, which doubled them. The stress of illness doubles them anyway, so mine were quadrupled. No wonder I wanted a drink! Supplementation of all the above deficiencies, including arachidonic acid, made a huge difference.

6. Genetic Flaws

I didn't want to go to genes, because as Bruce Lipton has proven, they don't have as much influence on us as we used to think they did. Alas, my trusty biofeedback machine has been telling me about mine anyway, and when I finally gave in and researched them, I saw they were important after all, because they have to do with immunity and blood and spleen in my case. In fact, I had a client recently who had the same two about immunity, which is uncommon, so I was surprised. My prominent one is hereditary spherocytosis. With this genetic flaw, your body makes your red blood cells in ovals instead of rounds, and your spleen mistakes them as foreign enemies and kills them, leaving a low count of red blood cells to fight infections like Lyme, etc. I find it necessary to take spleen glandular supplements for this as needed. I can tell from feeling pain in my right lower calf in the front above the ankle. This is a very good sign to be aware of. With my spleen making toast out of my RBCs that are oval shaped in Spherocytosis, my spleen is constantly overworked, and I don't want to wind up in the hospital having it removed, so I need to be aware of it's nature, along with my other organs.

I have other genetic flaws that involve immunity deficiency, sex-linked ones, and more, but I found almost no place to go for more information on the genetic flaws. The tests available are for particular illnesses, and they are very expensive. Besides, what can we do about "the luck of the draw"? I will say that things often show the "conception vessel" problems on my machine, and Mom told me that I was conceived at the height of my father's "drinking career," which may have something to do with it? Sounds like an old movie.

CHAPTER 6

Health Tidbits and Useful Tools

---

1. White Dove Healing Arts-(866-989-9342) www.whitedovehealing.com -

This leader in homeopathy is a family-owned enterprise started by Dr. Bill Cunningham when Professor Bill Nelson was inventing his first biofeedback machine and testing for frequencies. Cunningham and Nelson were friends, and the products my biofeedback machine shows as homeopathics on the client tests are available at White Dove Healing Arts for more protracted treatments. I have been ordering from them since I started my own biofeedback work fourteen years ago, and have been very happily served by them. What's more, their product Ameba-Fuge is the best thing I've been able to find in the United States today for amoeba infections. They also have Bacteria-Fuge and a host of other products. Now they've opened their Colorado store to the public, offering cell-phone neutralizers, shower filters, and Zeniral products. You can call for a catalog. Bill has taught many biofeedback classes and is an expert, as is his son, Jake. Look them up on YouTube and see for yourself. Ask Jake about the new Eductor biofeedback machine, too, Professor Nelson's latest biofeedback machine upgrade. Every medical professional should move into the incredible world of these unbelievably advanced health testers based on quantum physics.

2. Virapress Antiviral- (www.virapress.com, a division of Biostasis, Inc.)

Larry Griffin was a very sick guy who discovered his own cure and wanted to share it with the world. It's called Virapress. Thankfully, I found this product many years ago and spoke with Larry about Lymees using it. He was very informative and was working on its use on Dengue Fever in other parts of the world. With Zika now and other coming viruses, plus the flu and colds, I keep a stash of it on hand all the time. People don't realize that antibiotics don't fix viruses; they only help bacterial infections, and don't necessarily kill them, but may just drive them deeper. Virapress is for colds, flus, viruses.

At the first sign of anything like sneezing or chills, I gulp down some Virapress. I ask P how many I need—it's usually five—and by morning, the symptoms are almost gone, so I take a few more to keep it gone. I also take it for one of the Lyme coinfections that causes chronic fatigue, EBV, or Epstein-Barr Virus. In a day or two, my energy is all back to normal. This works for other Herpes, CMV, HH6, and so on that kept me in bed for years before I found Virapress. It prevents the Lyme relapses that were so devastating they took months to get over, severely weakening my body again. As a Medicare aged citizen, I haven't found a doctor via the supplemental health insurance programs who has ever heard of it, showing how large the gap is between our medical system and natural healing. Virapress uses interferon, a natural immunity addition. Add to this that these doctors don't speak English, and we have a cultural gap as well. The reason youth of today don't go to medical school to become doctors may stem from the results they see all around them and in their families—conventional medical techniques are clearly not working in todays complicated illness picture.

3. Nano sized Silver

Nano silver is small, particle-sized silver in deionized water, in suspension, much smaller than colloidal silver in suspension. They're in a nanosuspension or much more stable state.

I'd heard about nano silver, and when I ordered some online, I was thrilled by the results it showed me. The particle size is small enough to get inside a cancer cell and kill it, unlike colloidal or high PPM (parts per million) size that remain outside the cells. The potency yields a forty-times-greater per unit of silver, so there's a great advantage, plus the penetration into cells, capillaries, pathogens, and backwater body tissues. Also, it has the low PPM; I use one with 10 PPM. Only in the last few years has this technology come to boost immunity and fight pathogens with silver so natural to the body in our original blueprint. And because of it's low PPM, it doesn't destroy healthy stomach flora.

I can't say enough about having a supply of nano sized silver around all the time too, as it's the silver that will work on bacterial infections, fungal infections, and topical infections. It's also great for lung infections. These are the staples everyone should know about so that they don't need to go to the doctor over common things anymore. As you take total responsibility for your own health, you take your power back. Each of these truth discoveries I put to use made me feel more erect, and I became the master of my own fate again. A miracle indeed.

4. Phosphatidylcholine (Amino Acid)

I went to a DO or Doctor of Osteopathy, and told him my nerves were shot from all the stress and illness over a lot of years. He sent me home with phosphatidylcholine and directed me to take six capsules every night before bed, which equaled 12,000 mg. of choline every night—yes, 12,000 mg.—he said one couldn't take too much of it. He explained to me that the autonomic nervous system has two sides: the sympathetic nervous system, which is the fight-or-flight side, and the parasympathetic nervous system, which is the calm and steady side. I lived my entire life up until then in fight-or-flight mode, he said, and that choline would support the parasympathetic nervous system to balance my central nervous system and support it. He told me it would take a while at these high dosages and that we could reduce it over time but that I should always take it, as I still had many stressors that were overtaxing the sympathetic system. I was to take it before bed because it would also help me sleep more soundly.

This was another totally unheard of great success recipe for me, and I've been eight years on choline now, taking it as needed. Today I vary between three and six caps every other day if things are calm, and every day if stressors appear. I ask P how much I need. The prescription kind he gave me isn't online, but there are high-dose capsules available online that I use successfully—the higher the milligram count, the better.

I have a friend who writes great song lyrics and poetry, and sometimes he sends them to me for feedback. His work is very cool, but I noticed it always seemed tentative, not centered and grounded, and I told him the story of choline, and he said he was going to try it. A few months went by before I got some more lyrics, and all of a sudden, his work sounded rock solid, strong and secure, so I had to ask if he was taking the choline. And he said yes. I could tell, and when he sent more lyrics over the next few months, I suddenly got that tentative kind again, and I asked if he was still taking choline when he wrote it. He said he ran out, but now that I'd brought it up, he was going to get some more right away.

I keep reading more great things about choline, which is also a neurotransmitter. Phosphatidylcholine maintains cell structure, fat metabolism, memory, nerve signaling, and liver health, and it is a precursor to neurotransmitters. Called the "miracle molecule" for antiaging and weight loss, it is an essential phospholipid. Choline levels in cells decrease with age, and as it also helps skin elasticity, it really is antiaging.

This is not to be confused with lecithin, which is a mixture of several lipids, including choline and phospholipids. Choline is used for Alzheimer's, anxiety, manic depression, tardive dyskinesia, hepatitis, eczema, gallbladder disease, circulation, high cholesterol, PMS, and now nerves. What it has done for my nerves has made me feel whole and balanced again, not reactive or jumpy, and it does a lot for a good night's sleep. It adds to my confidence and sense of well-being.

I consider the three of these—Virapress, nano silver, and choline, to be staples in my home for all the reasons mentioned. Each of these gets big brownie points for keeping me in charge of my health instead of handing over the keys to pathogens. Knowledge is power all right, and knowing these products and what they can do for me has helped enormously to boost my confidence and set me free as my health returns and I feel it.

5. Bipolar/Manic Depression

These disorders are often a result of mercury poisoning, either from the fillings in your teeth or even inherited prenatally if your mother had dental work while she was pregnant.

6. Stomach-Acid Test for Heartburn

Swallow one tablespoon of apple cider vinegar or lemon juice. If the pain disappears, you have too little stomach acid, not too much.

If the pain gets worse, you have too much acid. Taking antacids is bad for you, and it's usually because you have too little acid, not too much that the symptoms of heartburn appear, so take this test if you take antacids.

7. MSG and Excitotoxins

The bad effects of MSG last long after you eat it. (See Dr. Blaylock's book *Excitotoxins: The Taste That Kills*.) Avoid all forms, including soy sauce—natural soy has MSG naturally.

8. Numbers on Produce

Read them! If it begins with an eight, it has been genetically modified. A first number of nine means it was grown organically with no pesticides.

9. Detoxing

Artichokes, cucumbers, asparagus, leeks, watercress are some good detoxers, and Dr. Clark's liver and gallbladder cleanse is great, which you can find online now as well as in her terrific books. Many products exist out there to help detox heavy metals, cleanse the colon, clear out Candida, detox the liver, kidneys, and bowel, and so on. Getting the cellular waste out of your body is essential for health—and for staying young. Vitalzym is a product worth the price for this. I detox all the time. I have been detoxing mercury for many years now and it still comes up on the machine. It's not in just one place in your body, it's all over you. Parasites and bacteria and viruses and fungi pathogens eat heavy metals and store them, so when they die, the metals are released again in your body, and can be detoxed or eaten by the next pathogens or their babies. The best way to stay young is to detox regularly, the liver, kidney, colon, heavy metals, bowel, skin, etc. Lyme gave me many dental caries when I was in my teens and had no sugar or sodas or sweets in my diet, because it wanted heavy metals for food!

10. Anticancer Defense

As Professor Nelson taught me, defending against cancer involves having enough minerals and fatty acids to protect us. Add antioxidants, detox, detox, detox, and radical forgiveness of self and others.

11. Parasites

The Center of Disease Control (CDC) discovered that the average American carries two pounds in total of three hundred different kinds of parasites, and they like the same food that cancer does: sugar, processed foods, junk food, fast food. I use Parasite Free, an all-natural product, to clean them out as necessary and take Hcl with every meal so they don't get in. Markus Rothkranz's website www.markusproducts.com is where to find Parasite Free. 1-888-517-3820. Markus is a huge health pioneer and has many products and other websites. However, one protocol does not fit all, as I have shown with the eat your greens example and Lectins, so ask your testers what is good for your own body as you search all the products out there on sites.

12. Melatonin and Sleep

It's best to sleep in a totally dark room so that the pineal gland will make its own melatonin. You'll need blackout shades, curtains, and a battery-run clock. Never have your clock radio on the nightstand next to your head, or cell charger, etc. If your pineal gland is not working still, there are supplements for the hypothalmus, which is also supported by taking lithium supplements. There are supplements of various kinds for pituitary or combinations too. Test to see if you need the hormone or glandular, etc.

13. Impacted Fecal Matter

With age, we store impacted fecal matter in our colons. You may have heard that John Wayne was carrying fifty-six pounds of it when he died? Taking large doses of the excellent Wobenzym N proteolytic protein digesting enzyme on an empty stomach before bed will digest it all out in a few days. Dowse to determine how many for how long. I do twenty the first night and then reduce each night according to P. Pathogens and parasites feed on this so it's just another form of detoxing.

14. EMF Protectors for Cell Phones

Try a Total Shield device for office computers to flood the area with negative ions, or use Orgone pyramids, salt lamps, and so on. Kids should only use the text function of their cell phones. Don't use your cell phone in the car with kids, as the radiation bounces all over. There are several technologically advanced protectors available now online.

15. Power FX Silicone Bracelet

This little item also produces a flood of negative ions into the body, adding health and energy. When I take it off, I feel the difference, so I don't take it off anymore—even in the shower. It has two dots inside the silicone bracelet that face each other through the wrist and produce this bath of negative ions. I have been wearing mine for eight years now, and it still works great for such a modest cost.

16. Best Brown Rice Pasta

Tinkyada brand brown-rice pasta is the best gluten-free spaghetti, spirals, elbows, and penne ever, and all it is consist of is brown rice, rice bran, and water. It digests so easily and tastes better than pasta! Available in stores, on www.vitacost.com, or www.amazon.com.

17. Mycotoxins and Leaky Gut

Mycotoxins are the toxic excretions of fungi, and they can cause autoimmune diseases and disrupt oxygen and enzyme systems, leading to cancer. Mycotoxins from mold, fungus, and yeast make your hair fall out and give you nail fungus. They set up systemic shop inside you, creating leaky gut and making you crave carbs. Mycotoxins are found in stored grains and flour, yeast, nuts and seeds, corn, peanuts, cashews, grain-fed animals, antibiotic-fed animals, cereals, bread, cheese, white sugar, alcohol, mushrooms, and leftover foods after four days in the fridge. I know when I am craving sweets or carbs that either a parasite is behind it (some crave alcohol), or yeast, so I take my Yeast Management supplement. I would take this if I were going to drink wine or spirits made with yeast, or foods with yeast, before they set up the Candida spiral and you put on the pounds and can't control the cravings. It's not you doing it, it's them. That's why to say the Intro when testing, always, or they will give you the wrong answers to feed them.

18. Reverse-Osmosis Water or "R.O." water-

Don't drink it—unless it's only briefly for detoxifying. I drank it for two years, and it made me, along with my dogs, weaker and weaker. It's dead water and has nothing to give. Pure spring water, on the other hand, comes from rain going deep down into the earth, collecting memories along the way, until it resurfaces as "complete" water and is flammable because of its structure. Some health programs recommend it, I say not unless you are detoxing.

19. Accidents and Adrenals

Your adrenals are shot if you have enzyme depletion in your right and left hemispheres. Accidents make the adrenals toast and make a time shift—you get interfering patterns in your energy field (enzymes). If your adrenals are too weak, you can't relax. I had this on top of the Pyroluria muscle tension and inability to relax, Candida cravings, and stress. Only now with supplements am I able to relax after many years, like the choline and the deficiencies from Pyroluria, the yeast fighters, etc. Straightening out my chemistry is the only way I can return my health and thrive. That's why it's fun to find every aspect of the original blueprint of who you are for the whole picture as a Medical Detective par excellence!

20. Brain Test–Left and Right

Test if the brain is "off" on the left or right by having a person hum and see if they go weak, or count and go weak. If it's off on the right brain, humming will go weak, and on the left, counting goes weak. My machine will say "balance right and left brain" or "balance front to back", etc. Head injuries can do severe damage in many ways I learned.

21. Underground Geopathic Stressors

Dowse and check under your house for underground water veins, sewers, gray water lines, fault lines, paranormal interferences, radioactive geological matter, noxious resonance from mold/fungus, and additional Geopathic Stressors. It's important. These can really undermine your immune system and cause serious illnesses. If you have any of these I would consult a professional dowser. Also read up on which ones you find to see if you can mitigate it with professional Dowser's help. The Water Cross in my house was not fixable for example, but some are moved by the help of Orgone and other tools and devices, to offset the negative effects without having to move.

22. Natural Sugars

D-Mannose and D-Ribose are healthy, natural sugar supplements. D-Mannose works great for UTIs and D-Ribose for energy. I follow Dr. Stephen Sinatra's excellent book *The Sinatra Solution* for my heart and cardiomyopathy. where he tells all about the influences of D-Ribose. These are natural sugars our body needs. Sinatra's book is essential to my handling my heart's needs, especially with his basic combination of the amino acid Carnitine, D-Ribose, and CoQ10, which I take often. My biofeedback machine tells me when my heart is acting up, like the left ventricle, etc. Then I look it up in this Sinatra book for the best protocol treatments.

23. Soy

Say no to soy; its compounds block the absorption of nutrients and minerals like calcium, magnesium, iron, and zinc. It is also very processed, and it disables enzymes your body needs. It also blocks thyroid function and protein absorption. It is a phytoestrogen, and Dr. Clark linked it to breast cancer, and many others have agreed over time. People are allergic to it as well but don't know it. Don't eat soy-fed animals or eggs, which seem to include chicken, turkey, and even beef now, incl. free range animals. I'm told all commercial chickens are fed soy and corn today, which is why I became allergic to chicken as I mentioned.

24. Bitter Is Better

It heals and enlivens your liver. The best parasite remedies are the bit-terest. Parasite-Free I mentioned, along with Dr. Clark's well proven parasite program. Dandelion leaves, bitter gourd, go sour from sweet tastes. Over fifty we have less and less Hydrochloric Acid (Hcl) in your body naturally to kill parasites and I take it as a supplement to replace that. This is one of the most severe causes of aging in my mind, because it allows the parasites and amoebas to take us over with Candida and molds. Digestive enzymes are a must over fifty also so you get the nutrients into your body from food. Diseases set in oth-erwise, as do parasites, and you lose your energy and ability to heal. I say that your body is not your friend over the age of reproduction, so you have to take supplements to maintain it. So dump sweet for sour!

25. Fruit with Seeds

Don't eat seedless fruits, as they can be hybrids with high sugars and low nutrients and messed up genetically. Finding good food is getting harder and harder as we continue to deplete the soil, use pesticides and herbicides, drop aluminum and barium on the earth.

Growing your own if you can is the best answer, or trading. I find Farmers markets very expensive, usually not organic, and who knows what is in the soil they use. Living in Las Vegas, the earth there was contaminated from testing above ground for many years. Ask your energy testers! If you dig them, take P to test what you want to buy first. "From 100% pure light, show me what foods on this table are good for my body."

26. Plastic Bottles–The Right Numbers to Use
Plastic water bottles that do not leach plastic into your water are #2 HDPE, #4 LDPE, or #5 PP. Usually sold are #1, which is good for only one use. Say no to #7 altogether.

27. Fatty-Acid Deficiency
Feel cold all the time? It's probably a fatty-acid deficiency. All eighty-eight fatty acids are essential and protect you from viruses and cancers. Cooked oils are a slow poison, making cells porous. Uncooked, natural, cold-pressed olive oil is best. Be sure to dowse it before you buy it, as soy oil is being silently added to many oils to increase their shelf life—even when the label says "pure" olive oil, check it.

28. Carbonated Drinks
After one cola drink, your white-blood-cell count is reduced by fifty percent, and your immunity is shot for eight hours. Iced tea has antioxidants, and you can sweeten with Stevia. Be sure tea bags are not moldy when you make teas.

29. Malabsorption
Malabsorption can occur as a result of gluten sensitivity, lectins, or Celiac disease/Sprue, where the cilia in your intestines that absorb the nutrients flatten out so they can't absorb. Parasites, Crohn's disease, and other infections cause malabsorption as well, starving you

while the pathogens and parasites feast. Ask P if you have malabsorption of nutrients.

30. Chlamydia, Mycoplasma, Bartonella infections and the Heart

Heart patients should be tested for Chlamydia, Mycoplasma, and Bartonella, as they can cause serious heart infections. Because Chlamydia was labeled a sexually transmitted disease, it's never mentioned. Bartonella can cause atherosclerosis., like it did for me. *Chlamydia pneumoniae* is called the "heart attack germ." These are also Lyme coinfections remember, and I happen to have all three, so the Buhner books are a must read for these. Mycoplasma is present in 90% of patients with Rheumatoid Arthritis, and in 50% of cancer patients. It eats more nutrients from your tissues than any other infections due to it's small genome, and you must supplement for these nutrients if you have Mycoplasma. Energy tools to ask these questions can save your life, as these infections are almost unknown in conventional medicine, so untreated, and cause so much pain and suffering that can be avoided by proper natural treatments.

31. Nattokinase

Using aspirin as a blood thinner can have side effects—it is a salicylate that some, including me, are sensitive to. Nattokinase is a very good natural blood thinner that also dissolves clots. It is one mushroom that doesn't bother me. Foxglove is another natural blood thinner. The drugs for thinning blood are very toxic and need so much monitoring, are devastating in side effects and testing, I say no to them if I can use these.

32. Vitacost.com

www.vitacost.com has a nice selection of supplements—and nearly everything else. It is a real favorite for quality supplements that are a lot cheaper—without the overhead of health food stores, they can save you a lot. They also offer gluten-free foods like Tinkanyada, and have fast shipping.

33. Lyme Coinfections and Vitalzym

Coinfections of Lyme disease include Bartonella, Babesia (Malaria), Mycoplasma, Ehrlichia, Rocky Mountain Spotted Fever, Trench Fever, the Rickettsias, Legionnaire's disease, Encephalitis, Brucellosis, Chlamydia, all the Herpes groups (including Epstein-Barr virus, HH6, CMV, Zoster, etc.), West Nile virus, Scleroderma, many forms of mold and fungi, staph, strep, Candida, vertigo, chronic fatigue, MS, Parkinson's, heart palpitations, Bell's Palsy, allergies, multiple chemical sensitivity, brain fog, joint problems, excess fibrinogen, Pyroluria, chronic inflammation, acute respiratory illness, meningitis, collagen problems, anxiety, opiod deficiency, and edema. Also remember that all these entities poop, creating waste that is very detrimental to your health. I use Vitalzym to take out the waste or Wobenzym N to digest them out.

34. Degeneration/Regeneration

At any given time, your body is either degenerating or regenerating. I have found from my biofeedback results that I'm degenerating more when I'm not exercising and regenerating more when I am exercising, so just walking will do a lot to increase the energy that is necessary for healing and put the body in a regenerating mode.

35. Peelu Digestion Gum

Peelu chewing gum with xylitol is good for digestion and gingivitis. I can't digest xylitol so I don't take other products using it, but this one is handy and fun.

36. Cold Drinks

Cold drinks with ice at meals or after meals will slow down your digestion and solidify food. This reacts with acid and will line the intestine, where it will turn into fats that can lead to cancer. It's better to drink hot soup, tea, or warm water after a meal (maximum of four ounces). No more than a cup of liquid should be taken with a meal, so when you place your food orders, don't order big gulp sizes or your digestion will be toast. I wonder why food servers think they are doing you a favor with refills after refills. We forgot the basics.

37. Molds and Brain Damage

Molds can mimic brain damage such as a concussion or brain injury, causing symptoms from depression, memory loss, seizures, paralysis, tics, and spasms to loss of balance, slow reaction time, learning disabilities, poor attention, emotional problems, Autism, and schizophrenia. Molds can travel across the globe. Mycotoxins are among the most potent carcinogens.

38. Harmful Chemtrails

Tinnitus and more can be caused by chemtrails in the United States and NATO allies from government planes adding aluminum oxide, barium, mycoplasma, anthrax, molds, fungi, and so on into the atmosphere. More information is available at this website: www.stop-sprayingcalifornia.com.

39. Drugs–Prescribed or OTC

Say no to drugs, both prescribed or over the counter, except for emergencies. Start learning about herbs, natural cures, all in the health food stores. Sprouts, Natural Grocers, Whole Foods, etc. can change your life. Drugs have not only contaminated the ground water, but they have contaminated our bodies, that can't even recognize them so can't dispose of them. They ruin your detox pathway organs, the liver and kidneys, by collecting there. Detox them all out and stop putting them in. There is a natural remedy for almost everything except emergency situations or conditions. Say no to all drugs, over the counter drugs too. Keep Virapress around for colds and flu, Echinacea and Goldenseal for bacterial, P'au de Arco for fungal and bacterial, etc. etc. *Prescription for Nutritional Healing* by Balch is a good place to start looking for natural remedies.

40. Ingredients in Gluten-Free Products

Beware of ingredients in gluten-free products, like sugar, that can still cause weight gain and high blood pressure. The website www.tastespotting.com has some recipes under "Gluten-Free" that are far superior. I'm doing a lot more cooking at home nowadays, tired of finding GMOs, insecticides, food additives and dyes, preservatives, soy oils, and so on in my test results. When I eat out, even at the top restaurants, I take my lectin blockers (2) before I order or ten minutes before I eat.

41. Walking Pneumonia

Walking pneumonia, the popular term for *Mycoplasma pneumoniae*, creates reactive oxygen free radicals that modify the RNA and DNA of cells, which can lead to malignant transformation. Nearly 90 percent of certain late-stage cancers show that it makes them more malignant and metasticizing, also causing vasculitis, so don't just "live with it." Stephen Harrod Buhner's book on Mycoplasma and Bartonella is excellent in how to deal with these awful coinfections of Lyme. Mycoplasma steals the most nutrients of any pathogen, especially fatty acids, which you recall Dr. Nelson says protects you from cancers. His basic protocol is using Cordyceps, Chinese skullcap, Isatis, Houttuynia, N. Cysteine, Vitamin E, and olive oil. Depending on what symptoms you are experiencing, he has the things to add for them. He also has diet recommendations like lots of Pomegranate juice all day. He has an immunity formulation to help as well.

42. Low Hydrochloric Acid (Hcl) and Digestion

Low levels of Hcl is associated with Celiac disease, bloating, a too-full feeling after meals, weak nails, acne, iron deficiency, parasites, undigested food, and gas. It is common in chronic Candida, asthma, hepatitis, autoimmune diseases, rheumatoid arthritis, Lupus, diabetes, food allergies, gastritis, Graves' disease, pernicious anemia, osteoporosis, psoriasis, thyrotoxicosis, hypothyroid, and vitiligo fungal disease. For me, taking betaine Hcl with meals has been essential for digestion, absorption, and overall health.

43. A Pregnant Mother's Foreign Cells

When a woman is pregnant, the blood of both the mother and baby has dozens of "foreign" cells and DNA besides those from each parent. They are likely to be from siblings of the parents or the parents' parents. There is a sieve between mother and the in-utero baby, a passage of cells between generations. I learned this on my favorite television show, *Through the Wormhole*, hosted by Morgan Freeman.

So your children who resemble your brother or sister or grandmother or grandfather have cause.

44. Canola Oil

Canola, also known as rapeseed, is the most toxic of all food-oil plants—its oil depresses the immune system. It's still used because it's cheap, not because it's healthy. It fills the shelves of the health food stores today, and nobody knows better. Until now. Avoid it.

45. Childhood Ear Infections

Childhood multiple ear infections can be fixed with chiropractic treatment and should not be treated with antibiotics ever. Lungworm (in dogs) and roundworm exist in over eighty percent of chronic fatigue patients. Lyme also causes it, and other things like Epstein Barr Virus (EBV).

46. Iodine Deficiency

Iodine deficiency can contribute to breast cancer, and it is deficient in most of us now that they've taken it out of bread. I squirt Lugol's Iodine into a glass of whatever I'm drinking—water, fresh juice, whatever—and ask P if I'm deficient and whether I should do that three times a day or every other day, and so on. An ounce of prevention is worth a pound of cure.

47. Mold–Spices, Juices, and Brown Rice

Beware of mold in common spices in jars. Brown rice is brown from mold; after cooking it, add vitamin C to kill the mold, stir it in, and it will be okay. All fruit juices in bottles except pineapple and mango are moldy shortly after opening.

48. Taking Responsibility

Kicking stress out my back door, creating boundaries and maintaining my field, detoxing negative emotions that hold onto illness, and becoming one hundred percent responsible for my health and my imprint on this earth was a tall order for me. With each rung of the ladder of truth, I gained a lot of self-respect out of awareness. I was raising my level of consciousness every day and didn't need to explain it to anybody. I just honored my truth tools and truth teachers, and calibrated people places and things, relationships, business, policies, and health questions. Self- reliance is a spiritual value I continue to improve.

49. Household Cleaners

Use baking soda or vinegar and water as household cleaners—no more, no less—and you won't be adding more toxins to your home. The blue in Windex is a toxin, who needs it. Clorox must be abandoned for good in any usage as it contains so many toxins and poisons it has already effected our water supply and many other areas. It should be banned as a toxic waste. There are NSF bleaches available that do not cause this at the supermarkets, look for the initials NSF.

50. The Heart Association's Margarine Mistake

Never eat margarine—it suffocates your cells. Recommending it is a mistake the Heart Association never corrected. Check all the health associations to see who supports them, and you will see why cures are never found. Most of the "Associations" of health are paid for by drug manufacturers and don't ever find cures. I wonder why.

51. Soy-Free Eggs

The chickens we eat are fed soy now, and so are some cows, so I have to look for soy-free eggs in health-food stores like Natural Grocers, Sprouts, and Whole Foods. I'm allergic to soy, and so are a lot of people are who are not Asian. So is my dog, so I now have to hunt down chickens that weren't fed soy. Got any?

52. The Problem with Wheat

Wheat is the most addictive food on the planet. Despite this, people will go to war to protect their croissants—which proves that very point. Your favorite foods are usually the ones you're allergic to. It may be okay to give it a "time out" and ask P when you can eat it again in order to quell the allergic inflammatory reaction.

53. Natural Healing Practices

There are hundreds of natural healing practices, called many things. Complimentary, Integrative, Alternative, and Energy Medicine are Holistic kinds of Medicine. There are Chiropractors, Natural Doctors, and all kinds of hands-on practices as well as Massage and Bowen and so many more. Allopathic doctors don't learn natural healing, or nutrition, or whole body treatments, and they prescribe drugs for remedies instead of natural herbs and such. They also are one of the most dangerous sources of mistakes, along with hospitals. I try and stay away from both. Find the best resources nearest you and try them all. It will open your mind and heal your body as you learn to find people who really care and have a lot more time for you than normal MDs, who give you fifteen minutes and an Rx.

54. Don't Be a Turkey

I feel turkey-ed to death already—it's so prominent as a health food today. I don't get energy from it, so after the chicken and soy story, I found out that turkeys are being given food additives like beer, pain relievers, antihistamines, antidepressants, arsenic to prevent disease, and—you guessed it—soy and corn. Martha Rosenberg's book *Born with a Junk Food Deficiency* adds that these turkeys are at risk from sudden death from heart, pulmonary edema, weak bones, and lesions. You want that for lunch?

55. Deficiencies can be Causing Heart Arrhythmias

Heart arrhythmias can be caused by simple deficiencies in selenium, potassium, magnesium, calcium, vitamin E, folic acid (B vitamin), CoQ10, or the amino acid L-carnitine. Over my fourteen years with my biofeedback machine, I've had arrhythmias many, many times. Since malabsorption was a problem regardless of my diet or the supplements I took, pathogens (bacteria, viruses, fungi, parasites) eat your nutrients, vitamins, minerals, etc. I would test on the EPFX/SCIO, and it would show these deficiencies as acute, and I would take the supplement. If I wasn't due to use the machine, I just asked P which of the above list I needed and did it that way. It's such an uncomfortable feeling, I appreciated being able to fix it quickly if deficiency was the cause. Infections can cause this as well. Since heart arrhythmias are so frightening to feel, I try and look for the deficiencies first for relief where I find it fastest. Usually it is deficiencies in one or more of these.

56. Thermography

Thermography should be used in place of mammograms, which can cause cancer. Thermography can also show other body hotspots and is preferable to X-rays, MRIs, CAT scans, and other methods that expose you to radiation. And for all their claims about digital X-rays being better, the radiation still showed up on my machine, making my positive magnetic number higher than the negative number when it should be lower. This can add to cancer causes. I am detoxifying radiation now, and if you had a lot of radiation, you should too.

57. Ultrasound

Ultrasound is another radiation-free testing method that can be used successfully and not harmfully. It is used in many ways and should be available with the right Wellness Practitioner offices, so seek them out.

58. Weakness of Cancer Cells

Cancer cells are very weak, and in order to take over, the patient's cells must be even weaker. So, as per the Yuen Method to strengthen weaknesses, that's our goal. I eat a very healthful diet, but my malabsorption problems, genetic flaws, and host of freeloading pathogens have given me a very weak system and lowered immunity as I aged, which I am working to reverse now. I had to eliminate stress, though a major contributor, up my nutrients, even via vitamin injections, and eliminate EMFs and toxins—and the rest was easy! Joke. Okay, bad joke.

59. Natural Fabrics

Only wear natural clothing. Cotton, silk, and wool are beneficial because they conduct electricity, and our bodies run on electricity.

Children raised wearing synthetics can become prone to allergies. A half-and-half polyester-cotton blend will conduct half the electricity of pure cotton. Bedding should be one hundred percent cotton, and you should skip the feather pillows. Even though feathers may be natural, they cause severe allergic reactions in a lot of people, including me.

60. Papaya Seeds and Parasites

Because papaya seeds contain arsenic, eating them will help kill parasites. Eight to ten seeds will do. I learned this when I lived in Mexico and saw the natives doing it. Walnuts and figs and pumpkin seeds also help with parasite control, as to a great extent does taking Hcl with meals.

61. GMO Food in Restaurants

Avoid GMO (genetically modified) food. I didn't know that a lot of restaurants use GMO foods, especially chain restaurants and fast-food restaurants. (Some are changing this practice now, as I see on TV.) Another reason I'm enjoying cooking food at home more now is because I know what's in it. No more mystery ingredients and GMOs.

62. Negative Energy in Metals

Metals collect negative energy, so beware of anything besides 18 karat gold or higher. Gold with a lower karat rating has too many alloys that attract negative energy. Sterling silver (it must be sterling only), pure copper, platinum, or stainless steel are okay. Avoid metal roofs, costume jewelry, and metal furniture. And we all know what aluminum does, right? It doesn't collect negatives—it collects your memory, so avoid anything made of aluminum, including cooking pots, aluminum foil, etc.

63. Perfumes and Hydrocarbons

Perfumes are made from hydrocarbons now, not oils from flowers, and they are made on the same chemical factories on Highway 10 in New Jersey that make the chemicals they add to make hamburgers taste like hamburgers in fast-food restaurants. Natural oils will do for scent. Highway 10 is lined with chemical factories of every flavor.

64. Fat

Eat fat to lose fat, but only from organic sources—pasture raised beef, soy-free chickens, and so on—because the ones fed antibiotics and hormones and pesticide laden vegetables store these substances in their fat. Our brain is seventy percent fat, so we need *healthy* saturated fats in our healthy diet, pure olive oil, butter, etc. Low-fat diets actually make you fat. Dr. Atkins said lamb fat is the best for your heart, and lambs from Australia or New Zealand eat cleaner food than lambs do here. The heart muscle operates entirely on fat, and so does the brain. No trans fats please.

65. Chlorine Bleach

Never use chlorine bleach (Clorox) on anything for any reason. It is highly toxic and loaded with dyes, heavy metals, and other harmful elements. It has already compromised our ground water because at one time we didn't know any better. The National Sanitation Foundation has approved a bleach that can be used safely and effectively, and it is available in all stores. If you can't find it, demand it. I know this is the second time I listed this, but I want you to remember it!

66. Ice Cream and Benzene

Ice cream can have benzene in it, a residue of the solvent used to clean its container. By government regulations, anything in packages, bottles, or containers has to be cleansed, but they don't say to cleanse the toxic solvent afterward, so it's often left in the packaging and doesn't have to be listed as an ingredient. Dr. Clark has proven the huge role of solvents in cancers, combining with particular parasites to cause different types of cancer. Isopropyl alcohol is a major one, as is benzene, and there are others. You need to check all cosmetics, shampoos, lotions, cleansers, and anything you use on your body or to put into it, including all supplements, food enhancers, ketchup, mustard, and so on for solvents. I found that more than half the many brands of supplements out there use solvents to clean the capsules before they get filled with vitamins. (I followed Dr. Clark's suggestion to freeze them to fix the solvent issue, and it worked.)

67. Digestive Aids

I take digestive aids because I need them. That includes Hcl, and Digestive Enzymes, and a good Probiotic. Pineapple and papaya work well as digestion aids, and so do apples. A slice of lemon or citrus in drinks or on food creates citric acid, which also helps digestion. Hcl and digestive enzymes in supplements can help too, and probiotics—very good quality and very strong, varied strains—are a must to prevent yeast and other infections in the gut. Yogurt is only beneficial in "plain" flavor and in small doses for acidophilus, because it's all calories otherwise and high in lectins. Entirely overrated in my opinion, like dessert.

68. Packaged Gluten-Free Breads and Mold

Store fresh-baked gluten-free breads or baked goods in the freezer, and you won't see that mold that forms right after baking, and all packaged breads from grocery stores show mold upon purchase.

69. Stainless-Steel Cutlery

Use only stainless-steel cutlery, as others leach out a lot of nickel. Chopsticks are good, and heavy-duty plastic cooking utensils are, too.

70. Microwaving Liability

Here's another word on microwaving and electromagnetic irradiation of microwaving reverse polarity over one billion times a second. Even in the low-energy range of milliwatts, no atom molecule or cell of any organic system can withstand such destructive power. Molecules are forcefully deformed, their quality impaired. The resulting new radiolytic compounds are unknown to man and nature. These impaired cells become easy prey for viruses, fungi, and other pathogens. Be sure not to eat microwaved food in restaurants either, as they nuke theirs, too.

71. Hydrogen Peroxide

Put a sprayer into a tall bottle of hydrogen peroxide and use it for cleaning. You can also use lemon as the natural bleach for mold around tubs, and water, of course, is the best solvent of them all, look at what it did for the Grand Canyon. Now that's a solvent.

72. pH balance

pH balance must be maintained at a neutral level. Too acidic makes acidosis and can feed pathogens that fuel disease. Meats and grains are acidic whereas fruits and vegetables are alkaline. So, if you have a roast beef sandwich, two acids are present, so you need a side of coleslaw and maybe a pickle, and add a lettuce leaf to the sandwich. Stress causes acid too, so eat alkaline food if you're stressed—and don't drink alcohol, because that's acidic too.

73. Barbecue Risks

Say no to barbecue. Lighter fluid is very toxic, as are the chemicals in briquettes. Carbon on burned or charred food is very carcinogenic too. Flames on meats, even in the broiler, are still bad. So even if you use natural woods the flames scathe the meats.

74. Long Labels

If labels on food packaging have more than six or seven ingredients listed, don't buy the product. Beware of the term "natural" on a label because it is misleading—it may not be natural at all. MSG is natural too, but it's one of the worst things you can eat. See Dr. Perlmutter's book *Excitotoxins*.

75. Light Skin and Zinc Deficiency

If you were born with very light skin as a Caucasian, you probably have a zinc deficiency, not a Cinderella complexion. Zinc is a very important mineral in enzymes and immunity. Don't worry—you won't change color by using zinc supplements! It is very important in immunity, production of enzymes, etc., so be sure you have your zinc.

76. Indoor Plants and Mold
Indoor plants grow mold that gives off spores. These get into your home's duct system and everywhere else, so I leave my plants outside and use a quality air cleaner inside.

77. Fungal Foods
Don't eat fungal food (yeast, mold, and so on) like bleu cheese, mushrooms, all grains and cheeses, wine and spirits made with yeast, or fermented foods. Hidden molds can exist in vitamins and such made with the Aspergillus process, soft drinks, fruit juices, peanuts, soybeans, Brazil nuts, and pistachios. The largest living entity on the planet is a mile-wide fungus in Michigan, if that helps.

78. Foods with Gristle
Eating foods with gristle, like lamb shanks, oxtails, Chinese dim-sum chicken feet, and pot roast has kept me free of arthritic pains by supporting the cartilage in my body. I learned that from my grandmother. Also eat organ meats, sweetbreads, liver, and gizzards. Mexican menudo, which is made from the stomach lining of cows, is also delicious. We need organ meats.

79. Low VOC Paints
Don't use petroleum products in any form, like Chap Stick. Latex is highly allergenic, so only use SafeCoat paints with low VOCs to re-paint and reduce toxic gas coming off the new coat. Don't put a baby in a just painted room! Don't use wallpapers or anything with toxic glues either.

80. Artificial Nails and Polish

Artificial nails and polish are very toxic. Look at the moons on your fingernails to see your oxygen level (not the pinky finger). If there's no moon in the thumbnail, check for cancer. Your nails show your diet deficiencies, especially the minerals. I like to read mine like a good information source.

81. Fluoridated Water

Fluoride in water or toothpastes, or animals that drink fluoridated water on farms where they came from, should be avoided completely. Use a shower filter for chlorine removal, and filter tap water throughout the whole house.

82. Pure, Organic Cream

Pure, organic cream is very healthy, and it takes fat to burn fat, so this is a good fat. Only eat organic, as pesticides can have a cumulative effect. As a prime example, note how the bee population is collapsing from the cumulative effect of pesticides.

83. Self-Cleaning Ovens

Self-cleaning ovens can kill pet birds and sicken pets, so be sure to remove them before you begin to self- clean your oven. Kids too. Be sure to open the windows and turn on fans.

84. A Shaker for Powdered Vitamin C

Getting a jumbo salt shaker to hold powdered vitamin C is an excellent adjunct for the table to sort of clean your food. This is a recommendation from Dr. Clark. Vitamin C can purify all the food on your plate. Use with brown rice, always, after cooking.

85. Cold Cereals

Cold cereals are among the worst foods to eat. Solvents are used to stick them together, they are moldy, grains are very allergic, they are highly processed, and they contain fluoride. For more information, watch the DVD *Let the Truth Be Told*.

86. Vitamin C Supplements

I have found little to no vitamin C in oranges from either Florida or California any longer. Those articles and the FDA lists must have been taking samples fifty years ago. In addition, orange juice produces wood alcohol, a solvent, and it is loaded with sugar. So, supplement vitamin C in your diet as high as you can tolerate it, and get it from kale or cantaloupe.

87. Grapefruit and Kidney Stones

Grapefruits are also low in vitamin C now, plus they give you kidney stones if eaten regularly, like I did in the mornings. Even tangelos are low in Vitamin C now, how grim.

88. Sugar Cravings and Chromium Picolinate

If I get big sugar cravings, I check chromium picolinate to see if I'm deficient in that important mineral. Deficiency in chromium and vanadium contributes to diabetes, and they are also sold in combination. I ask P how many I need while holding the chromium picolinate bottle, and it's usually a lot, like twenty. The next day, I ask again, and may need a few more or perhaps none. If P says I'm not deficient in it, I look for pathogens that make you eat—parasites, fungal infections like Candida, even ulcers make you crave food to feel better. Infections can make you feed them too.

89. Maximum Number of Supplements per Day

I take strong and natural (not synthetic) multivitamins (minerals, amino acids, etc.) and antioxidants daily because they cover what our foods can't provide any longer. Minerals are what make vitamins work. Dr. Klinghardt originally recommended taking no more than 10 capsules a day, but he bumped that up to 20 because ten wasn't enough. I've taken a lot more than that, but eventually my stomach protests. I know that Dr. Nick Gonzalez's great success with pancreatic cancer patients was due to heavy supplementation, up to 250 a day. Remember the story about the weak cells.

90. Aspartame and Sugary Sodas

Avoid carbonated sodas—regular *and* diet. The diet ones use aspartame, and the highly acidic pH of just one soda takes hours for your body to neutralize to the right pH. To do so, it draws on all your minerals, mostly from your bones. The sugary sodas are highly acidic too. Any artificial sweeteners are bad news, so use Stevia. Agave isn't so good either though it's less volatile than sugar on the glycemic index, but better than white sugar. I have noticed my body has different reactions to different sugars, like turbinado, brown sugar, etc. It's a good exercise to test your sugar reactions. White sugar is out the door for everyone though, along with white flour and white rice.

91. Precut Lettuce

Lettuce and other fruits and vegetables lose their nutrients as soon as they are cut up, so salad bars are deceiving, and precut salads in restaurants are no better. Lettuce is also in the ragweed family—just an FYI if you have allergies.

92. Deterioration in Food Quality

It takes eighty cups of today's supermarket spinach to give you the same level of iron you got from one cup fifty years ago. Similarly, it takes nineteen ears of today's corn to achieve the nutritional benefit of one ear back then. So we must supplement sufficiently.

93. Synthetic Supplements

Never buy synthetic vitamins. Vitamin B-12, for example, is made from sewer sludge stabilized with cyanide. The term "organic" only applies to foods, not supplements—and going organic is the best way to get the maximum health benefits of food today. Use solvent-free supplements, not made from aspergillus, yeast free.

94. High Histamines

High histamines and allergies may be reduced by taking L-methionine, the natural amino acid that oxygenates the liver, along with quercetin, which is in onions or supplements. Say no to drugstore antihistamines made of chemicals.

95. Alcohol and Yeasts

Alcohol, beer, and wine are made with yeasts and feed yeasts and Candida. Alcohol is also a solvent, encouraging microbes to nest instead of pass through. Alcohol is also a direct form of sugar into the bloodstream, which feeds pathogens like parasites and cancer, and all infections, too.

96. Moldy Foods

Bouillon cubes or powdered spices are very moldy. Make your own soup stock. Make gravy using the vegetables and onions you cook with a pot roast, pureeing them in a blender, and it will be tastier and a lot more nutritious than adding flour. Avoid black iced tea as it binds stools. Molds (fungus, yeast) can grow on virtually any substrate, including food, jet fuel, paint, rubber, textiles, electrical equipment, glass, stainless steel, dirt, and grease. Candida can go into your lungs, brain, heart, gut, and spleen, too. Detox it.

97. Disease Agents

Disease agents are PCBs, heavy metals, isopropyl alcohol, benzene, other solvents, asbestos (used in supermarket conveyor belts at checkout), azo dyes, parasites, fungus, yeast, mold, and bacteria. Use your ozonater to clean foods.

98. Fluorosis

Skeletal, tissue, and dental fluorosis are becoming common today as communities are forced to fluoridate their water supply. It's killed horses, dogs, and people. Chronic fluoride poisoning from this waste product of fertilizer must be addressed. Now, with a new president, we have hope that changes will be made. Mercury, still used in amalgam fillings, mining operations, and so on, that is put into the air without limits or penalties must be addressed also. As we improve our health through all the truth tools and books, and as our power returns, we can make changes.

99. Shock

Shock, whether physical or emotional, drains the adrenals, fatty acids, vitamin C, and the B vitamins from your body. Since the auto crash I had in 1973, I have been deficient in all these, and my adrenals don't improve by taking adrenal supplements. Forms of Shock, like Insulin Shock, or Hypovolemic Shock, and others, plus traumas, have extraordinary effects on the body and health, and must be identified, as per Dr. Hamer's work. Think about what unexpected and unresolved shocks you had in your life and resolve them now.

100. Shoulder Disease

Too many "shoulds." My machine tells me this too!

101. Detox Only When Strong Enough

Do not detox a body that is too weak, or nothing will move out of you. Build yourself up first so that you will be able to detox. This can take a while, and require energy making supplements and diet, and light exercise. You can go into a tailspin if you detox a body too weak to respond. I had a doctor giving me mercury detox IVs that made me so sick, and I would tell him it made me drink, and he said "well, everyone responds differently".

Now I see that I was too weak to be going through those multiple IV's then, and it nearly killed me.

102. Sinusitis

Sinus congestion? That's likely from a fungal infection behind the nose. I use Physicians' Standard Nasal Clear D-54 spray that has a little nose insert tube. This product has balanced oils, amino acids, and minerals to flush out the throat, nasal passages, and sinuses.

Used to improve the health of these areas so that infections don't go there, this is better than just killing pathogens. See www.physiciansstandard.com (949-407-8822). In about three weeks, the sinuses will be clear, and they'll stay clear for a long time. It has a little sting as your nasal passages return to health, so don't be alarmed.

103. Gout
Got gout? Herbal Shepherd's Purse before meals comes in drops or capsules. It is used for other things as well, but it's widely available and helps prevent gout. I gave myself a big gout attack using Glycine supplements for my muscles. So don't make the same mistake if you have gout, avoid the foods that set it off.

104. Spleen and other Glandular Supplements
I've already told you the signs of spleen problems showing up in pain in the right leg lower front of the calf, and how taking spleen glandular supplements I get online have made the pain go away and supported my spleen. There are many other "glandulars". I take some for "female" and some for "multi", for various organs, whatever body part is in need of a boost. With these gram negative bacterias like Mycoplasma, Lyme, etc., who knows where they are lunching on us. Learning the Anatomy is very helpful for knowing what you are feeling where and why, so you can identify the problem, and verify it with P. and the energy testers.

105. Nighttime Wakefulness
Do you wake up every night at the same time? I do. Sometimes it's between twelve thirty and one thirty, and I know from a Chinese medicine chart that my gallbladder is a likely cause. I ask P and if it's that, I

take three or four Standard Process A-F Betafood tablets and get back to sleep. If it's between three and five, my liver's the culprit, and I take Himalaya's LiverCare to get back to sleep. Sometimes it's choline I need, too. I ask P. which to take, and how many, and if it's all I need. Some women sleep with their husbands; I sleep with P and a small dog.

106. Amoebas/Protozoa

For weak immunity, use Ameba-Fuge from White Dove Healing for Amoebas. Test mullein leaf tea, coconut water, garlic, oregano oil (two to three drops plus juice of one lemon in water three times a day), neem juice (one teaspoon twice a day), beetroot juice, turmeric, mustard oil, papaya seeds (about eight at a time for low arsenic), pomegranate, vitamin C, zinc, black tea, and pumpkin seeds. Low lgA from chronic stress drains immunity and adrenals making elevated yeast dysbiosis, food allergies, IBS, Candida, Crohn's, Colitis and Autism, viruses, protozoa, parasites, and bacteria. To raise lgA, use colostrum and beta-glucans. Make your choices by asking which are good for you, since some may be phenols, lectins, salicylates, that you have a problem with so should avoid.

107. Colostrum

For immunity, use three capsules three times a day for a big boost and three capsules once a day for prevention. This is the first immunity from mother's milk.

CHAPTER 7

Miscellaneous and Conclusion

You may wonder why I didn't say more about Lyme disease, but I don't really need to here. Yes, it's epidemic and incredibly complicated, but as you have seen in my story, I had other things involved. We all do. I noticed through monitoring my health with my biofeedback machine for the fourteen years I've had it that the body is in a continual state of change, and every part of it is involved in that change. Lyme details, next book.

I saw many illnesses pop up on my tests over these years that scared me because of my image of "diseases" from Western/allopathic medicine. We were taught in using the EPFX/ SCIO biofeedback machine that if breast cancer shows up on a client's test, that doesn't mean she necessarily has it, but she is going in that direction. They said that if you are treating a client weekly, and the breast cancer comes up ten times, then likeliness is they have it. Unfortunately, allopathic medicine doesn't discover cancers until late in the game, at which point they are much harder to treat and cure.

I saw Lupus come up for me several times but not consecutively, and I zapped it to scramble its frequency until it stopped coming up. I also had MS show up consecutively for a whole year, which really frightened me because my fingers had been starting to twitch. But I told myself that if I go to the doctors, they'd give me drugs, and I'd be labeled for life and go downhill as a "victim" of the disease. Same with Lupus. I would have had to take their archaic tests, and they would nail the Lupus label onto me forever and give me more drugs. Many other ills showed up as well, but I just zapped away weekly, and they all went away. MS took a whole year, so it was the scariest, but I just didn't buy into it. I still have things like Parkinson's show up, and I just zap. These are typical of Lyme disease plus the multiple coinfections I have that attack me one at a time, as if taking turns. I'm sure these pathogens communicate and cooperate. As I've said, I've seen that by now, and they are connected to the miasms like one big, happy family of freeloaders that I keep under control.

If I'd gone to a regular MD, I'd have been diagnosed with one thing they'd call my "problem" when in fact there were many things. I was deficient in sulfur, let's say, and many other things. Lectins, which they wouldn't have found, are part of the whole picture that Western medicine never sees. I see only holistic MDs, naturopaths and alternative healers now.

I feel very fortunate that besides my biofeedback machine, I now have a host of alternative/ integrative/holistic/complementary resources at my disposal, like homeopathy, naturopathic doctors, chiropractors, massage, Bowen technique, Rolfing, yoga, acupuncture, Reiki, hydrotherapy, Chinese medicine, magnet therapy, Bach flower remedies, the Yuen Method, the Biomat, and meditation. They use no drugs or chemicals and work much better.

Western medicine, like my Western education, was all linear, while quantum physics has proven that the truth is holographic, not linear. My machine is based on quantum physics. I feel my tests are a lot more accurate than any I would get from an MD. That's why the MDs could never find anything wrong with me and told me it was "all in my head." As soon as I got my biofeedback machine, the proper test diagnosis was clear that it was Lyme disease, coinfections of Lyme, and much more.

People think parasites are only a problem in third-world countries, but they are wrong. I've had big problems with parasites, and I take Parasite-Free that I already mentioned, once a week for preventative maintenance. Holistic MDs have said that people are much sicker today with more complicated ailments. Recall the section on miasms where it states that this is in fact so. I think it's essential that for best health results, we now take over the job of being our own doctors and keep learning about truth tools to self-care in order to take back our health and take back our power, here and now.

I would have listed the *Townsend Letter* monthly magazine under "Truth Heroes," but it is more a compilation of (so far) unproven ideas and research on natural healing. It might be difficult reading for some, but I just kept reading it for ten years, and it started sticking. Some of the ideas in the *Townsend Letter* are new and exciting, and they were the first to start articles on Lyme disease and coinfections before any information was out there yet, so I am very grateful. The subscription rate is very reasonable, and I heartily recommend it for professionals or laymen.

I haven't discussed many of the important health factors, like water, or that love, tenderness, and concern increase its energy and stabilize it. Fear, aggression, and hatred reduce water's energy and destabilize it. See *Mysteries of Water* on YouTube. In *HEALTH & POWER*, I wanted to show you new tools I found to make a whole health protocol for everyone, as I already showed how one size doesn't fit all, and we have to be very flexible in changing our treatments as we notice changes in our bodies. Now, using your health tools, you can ask your pendulum all the right questions. You can ask P, "Do I have Lyme disease?" and get that one off your list, for instance. I used my P to read Brandon Bays' book *Journey*, and each time I felt an emotion when reading a passage, I asked P if I had an issue like that. I usually got a yes, because I started to well up reading her story, and that's a clue for sure. Then I put the book down and tried to remember what situation it might have been (especially in childhood, although not always). Something would pop up that I remembered, and I would use the Dowsing method to clear it, spinning the pendulum left to remove and then right to add positives back in.

I asked P for many things—never to hurt—but I could ask if business people were lying to me. Family, too. The power of learning to use these truth tools is so enormous that it can change your life, your health, your whole world, and your children's world. It has only been wrong a few times in twenty years because I asked a question the wrong way. Kinesiology is like intuition with clout. The more you do it, the sharper your intuition becomes. Never forget the Intro first. Our tools tap us into Universal Truth, available to each of us every day, anytime, all we need to do is ask. What a gift.

I also wanted to say in conclusion that words matter. What you say can change your DNA. Crime goes up in areas with the most swearing, and swearing attracts negative energy to the person doing it. We are all in this together, and we have to improve the global consciousness that covers our planet. I had to improve my aura strength and power with self-love and love of everything and everybody and stop my old ego's business power plays of trying to outsmart everyone and win, or the old me.

I look to Oprah for my role model. From her beginnings, her success now is from using the truth and God the source and sticking to those two things. She stayed as clear as possible from pitfalls and attackers, keeping her soul intact, staying with the truth and the Creator of all energy. I have never seen a person more honest with herself, showing every one of us among the millions out there the courage and determination possible when it is the truth that we are after.

I learned that I had to change. Change wasn't what we were taught—security was, which means we shouldn't change things, right? But my auric field is ever changing like my body, and I'm on a new adventure as a Medical Detective, asking P questions and using the Map of Consciousness to calibrate everything I allow in my field. The spiritual truth is that we are each responsible for everything that happens to us, because what we are aligned with vibrationally is what shows up. So, if we don't like what shows up, we have to change our vibrational frequency. It's a Buddhist tenet that our lives are just a journey of self-improvement, and I have followed that path out of necessity as much as choice, which is why I remind myself to sit on my ego the way Oprah does. It will always choose things that will not bring joy and happiness. When another's ego challenges mine, I feel my blood pressure start to rise, and I know I need to move out and away pronto. I remember Dr. Yuen's lesson about having no beliefs to defend, and it's easy.

I thank my readers, and I thank my teachers. God bless us all. I'll leave you with a poem I wrote:

BEE LOVE

If I were a little honeybee,
I'd sit on a branch of that far tree,
And let the wind sing a song for me,
While I enjoy the shade.

As the sun filled me with vitamin D,
I'd stop thinking what I'd like to be,
And feel the world just loving me,
Like Mother Nature made.

I'd fly about and suck some roses,
Stop and nap in little dozes,
And feel well fed and take my poses,
For all the world to see...

That I exist just as I please,
In nature's harmony, at ease,
Along with all the honeybees,
Who like to fly with me.

Who could expect an earth so grand
So bright as we go hand in hand?
In mirth and joy explore the land
With such delight I'd know,

That all God's creatures, large and small,
Have come with features keen to all,
To impress our teachers come next fall,
That will come to love us so...

Who look upon my little wings
And think of them as merry things,
That do my daily nectar job, which brings
The flowers back next year.

And when I'm coming close to done,
With all my chores this earthly run,
And have my last of all this fun,
I'll go with love, not tears.

—Andrea Smith Banks

ABOUT THE AUTHOR

Andrea Smith Banks grew up in the New York metropolitan area and attended the Barbizon School of Modeling at fifteen. After her graduation, she worked every summer as a fur coat model for a large furrier company on Seventh Avenue. Buyers flew into NYC in the summer to buy their furs for their fall market buyers around the country. Her employer thought she was in college, not high school. When the NYC Playboy Club opened, Andrea spent summers on 59th Street, working as a Playboy Bunny before going back to Syracuse University every year and receiving her BFA degree. Returning to NYC's Playboy for two more years after, Andrea later joined her mother's large real estate team in Clifton, New Jersey, as a Realtor. Her brother Eddy was a Realtor there also, and the two of them purchased some fixer-uppers to resell or rent. Andrea attended the Work of the Stock Exchange and Brokerage Office Procedure classes on Wall Street, along with other business courses, learning a lot about business instead of art now.

Always a voracious reader, Andrea took night classes in psychology at a neighboring school while still in high school. Her electives at Syracuse were Plato's *Republic*, and she became really hooked on studying philosophy, reading *The Conduct of Inquiry* while others her age were reading *Harpers* and *Elle* magazines. Her father's being an inventor made her curiosity unquenchable, although he had died unexpectedly at forty-six when Andrea was just twelve, a loss she felt her whole life.

Andrea married her college sweetheart, and they relocated to Las Vegas for his travel business. Andrea subsequently sold her interests in the real estate properties she owned back east with her brother, purchasing the Brown Derby Apartments in Las Vegas, built in the 1950s by Moe Howard of Three Stooges fame, a block from the Sahara and the Strip. Andrea owned these twenty-eight furnished apartments on almost an acre of choice property for twenty-eight years. They were her financial base, while resident managers lived on the property to handle the maintenance and tenants, and collect rents.

Meanwhile, Andrea was studying philosophy at the University of Nevada at Las Vegas (UNLV) as well as linguistics, semiotics, and sculpture. Her last philosophy class was one-on-one with the department chair studying epistemology, the theory of knowledge. In addition, Andrea maintained her career as a professional artist, painting in acrylics, mixed media, and drawings, with work shown in several galleries around the country as well as Las Vegas (see www.andreabanksartsandbooks.com). Her work is owned by Tom Cruise, Nicholas Cage, and other notable collectors world wide.

Andrea's husband had said to her, "I'll give you your toga and your lantern; you bring me back the honest man." He thought it was funny. They were divorced, and Andrea moved to San Francisco to start over. But a year later, Andrea suffered serious injuries in an auto accident while visiting her apartment business in Las Vegas. Andrea decided to move to Athens, Greece after a month long recovery at her mother's home in New Jersey. Her ex-husband knew she loved Greece and he was living there in his travel business there bringing in groups to Athens, so he brought her back to the seat of Philosophy where she stayed for two months before deciding to move there from San Francisco. She spent three of her happiest years in Athens before returning to Las Vegas to oversee her apartments and the managers, and take more classes at UNLV. Three years passed as Andrea healed and took care of business.

Next, Andrea went to seek a master's MFA degree in painting from the Instituto Allende in San Miguel de Allende, Mexico. She studied with James Pinto of Yugoslavia and also took advanced writing classes with known authors from Iowa State University. Pinto was like her adopted father, and he loved her talent and passion. Three years later, she was back in Las Vegas and her apartments, her financial hub. Issues with managers were often a problem; since all transactions were in cash, many helped themselves, until she found a wonderful couple from Iowa that she could trust.

Next, Andrea moved back to New York and the tony East Village to the American Felt Building on East Thirteenth Street to advance her art career, take classes like *Synapses of the Nervous System* at the New School of Social Research, and listened to CEO speakers from all the big corporations along with Rudy Giuliani. Andrea used the figure drawing models at Parson's for drawing exercise, and was often told by her classmates that she was the best of the best at drawing figures, always her forte. Andrea was glad to see her two favorite dance troupes again—Alvin Ailey and Twyla Tharp—and off-off-Broadway plays for inspiration of life in the creative hub of the Big Apple.

Back to Las Vegas after three years, she did more reading and classes, painting and overseeing the apartments, which were becoming part of a changing neighborhood now dubbed the "naked city." Keeping drug dealers out and the tenants safe became a full-time job, and even her Iowa managers would no longer live on the premises. The city made her tear down her apartments, hoping to collect this choice property, the single worst thing that ever happened to her in business. But she kept her property, now vacant land.

A year later, Andrea sold the Las Vegas land and looking for property to use for a new investment, and having such a bad taste from Las Vegas, she found commercial property in Prescott Valley,

Arizona. She also found a beautiful Prescott home with 360 degree views of the mountains and the charming small city. (She still also had her custom home in Las Vegas.) It was then that Andrea fell seriously ill. She felt like "the walking dead" now, and she could hardly get out of bed during her whole first year in Prescott, suffering from extreme fatigue. Andrea knew she had to do something, because even if the doctors didn't know what was wrong with her, she could still read in bed. Her mind was still sharp, if her body was failing and her energy went south. Through reading the books mentioned in *HEALTH & POWER* She became her own Medical Detective instead of giving in to pain and suffering as a way of life. Banks was always a veritable "information junkie." Ask her today what her strong suit is today, and she'll say, "Deciphering information." Eight years studying philosophy early on was probably the best training she could have had. Her friends and family think she's brilliant. Her dog? Not so much. Is she "driven"? Yes—driven to find the truth.

No one could give more insight finding the answers to taking your health back and taking your power back. Treating her Lyme disease's complexity and turning her health around from being among the "walking dead" to the vibrant, active life Andrea lives today is proof that she found the right answers—simple truths so easy to follow when you take back the helm of your life and health. Take back your health, and take back your power like she did—starting now. Recovery is learning how to manage Health issues smartly, one by one. The complexity of diseases today is not manageable with a half hour trip to the doctor anymore. Besides P, who is your best friend to healing? You.

It took Andrea Banks twenty years of experiences, trial and error, and studies, to amass this collection of valuable resources that work, and that everyone can use. For prevention or treatment, for your family or yourself, there is enough fantastic news you can use material for you to investigate over a very long time, using your copy of *HEALTH & POWER* and these truth tools. This exciting new adventure is one you can depend on forever, because Andrea Banks spent her life pursuing the truth and learning the tools to find it. It brings her great joy to share this with you, and invite you to the party.

CONSULTING SERVICES

Andrea Banks is available for consultation and may be contacted by email at www.andreabanksartsandbooks.com Her biofeedback testing is available and treatment for stress and relaxation. Professionals can get the details. Also, let Andrea know how you are using the information in this book for your own health recovery.

HEALTH & POWER book orders are available online at www.amazon.com using the title and author.

HEALTH & POWER copies are also available from the author's website: www.andreabanksartsandbooks.com, where you can see her paintings, drawings, and sculpture, and her contact information.

Printed in Great Britain
by Amazon

29011293R00095